DESIGN OF COMPILERS

TECHNIQUES OF PROGRAMMING LANGUAGE TRANSLATION

KAREN A. LEMONE

CRC Press
Boca Raton Ann Arbor London Tokyo

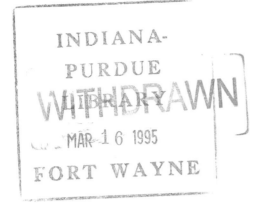
Acquiring Editor: Russ Hall
Production Director: Sandy Pearlman
Production Services: HighText Design and Production
Cover Design: Shi Young
Printing and Binding: Braun-Brumfield, Inc.

Library of Congress Cataloging-in-Publication Data
Lemone, Karen A.
    Design of compilers: techniques of programming language
translation / Karen Lemone.
        p. cm.
    Includes bibliographical references and index.
    ISBN 0-8493-7342-5
    1. Compilers (Computer programs).   I. Title.
QA76.76.C65L46   1992   91-29631
005.4'53—dc20   CIP

International Standard Book Number 0-8493-7342-5
Library of Congress Card Number 91-29631
Printed in the United States   2 3 4 5 6 7 8 9 0
Printed on acid-free paper

ABOUT THE AUTHOR

Dr. Karen A. Lemone is Associate Professor of Computer Science at Worcester Polytechnic Institute, Worcester, Massachusetts. She has been teaching compiler construction courses for over ten years and has served as interim department head of the Computer Science Department at Worcester Polytechnic Institute. She is currently a site-visitor for the Computer Science Accreditation Board (CSAB).

Dr. Lemone received her B.A. degree in Mathematics from Tufts University, M.A. degree in Mathematics from Boston College, and Ph.D. degree in Mathematics/ Computer Science from Northeastern University.

In the summer of 1985, she was invited as a foreign expert to Jilin University of Technology, Changchun, China. For the academic year 1988–1989, she was a *professor invité* at Ecole Polytechnique Fédèrale de Lausanne in Switzerland.

Dr. Lemone has published many articles in computing publications and has co-authored several books in computer science. She has been a reviewer for ACM *Computing Reviews* and IEEE *Computer*, as well as for conferences and various book publishers.

Her current research interests include semantic analysis and optimization techniques for object-oriented languages, applications of attribute grammars, and electronic document processing. She consults and conducts seminars in compiler implementation.

CONTENTS

4. Top-Down Parser Generators

5. Bottom-Up Parser Generators

6. Semantic Analysis and Attribute Grammars

7. Optimization: Introduction and Control Flow Analysis

8. Optimization: Data Flow Analysis

9. Optimization: Code Improvement

10. Code Generation Techniques

11. Production-Quality Compilers

12. Compiling for Special Architectures

Appendix A. Answers to Selected Exercises

Appendix B. Compiler Project SubAda

Index

PREFACE

The design and implementation of a compiler is an example of a large, complex programming project. Good compiler design and implementation requires the best knowledge of software engineering in order to handle the complexity.

The design and implementation of a compiler *text* is an example of a large, complex writing project. Good textbook design and implementation requires the best knowledge of educational pedagogy in order to handle the complexity.

There are many well-designed and well-implemented compilers today, which translate efficiently and are well modularized to deal effectively with the complexity of language translation.

This text, *Design of Compilers: Techniques of Computer Language Translation,* is modularized to deal with the pedagogical complexity of compiling. Principles are stressed whenever possible, with many, many examples to support and clarify these principles.

The standard phases of a compiler are discussed: lexical and syntax analysis are discussed from a compiler generator point of view. Chapters 1 to 5 are written to review the basic concepts as well as to describe the algorithms for *generating* scanners and parsers. Other topics include attribute grammars and their use in semantic analysis, algorithms and data structures for optimization and code generation, object-oriented languages, production quality compiler issues, and compiling for special architectures.

Although this book assumes some compiler background, it can be used in a graduate course which contains students with minimal to no background. Supplemental information may be provided on finite automata theory and symbol tables. Other compiler texts can be put on reserve for student reference. This book may also be used in a second undergraduate course. *Fundamentals of Compilers: An Introduction to Computer Language Translation* (by the same author) can be used in the first course.

There are two project choices. The simpler project implements a subset of Ada. This is described in Appendix B. The second and more difficult project choice implements PSOOL, a pseudo-object-oriented language.

Extensive reference lists are included at the end of each chapter. Graduate classes should be particularly encouraged to begin reading the literature.

This book contains a mixture of practical and (appropriate) theoretical information. I think students should be exposed to both. Language, grammar, and theoretical issues are discussed where they apply to compiling rather than in separate chapters so that students can see their relevance.

This book conforms to both the ACM and IEEE curriculum recommendations for compilers.

Possible course uses (*Fundamentals of Compilers: An Introduction to Computer Language Translation* is referred to here as Book I, while the present text is referred to as Book II):

- A full semester course (*easiest*): Book I: Simple exercises, omitting perhaps Chapter 5. Project: A recursive descent compiler (described in the addendum to each chapter) omitting Part V, the error handling routines of Chapter 6. Include Part IV even if Chapter 5 is omitted.

- A full semester course (*moderate difficulty*): Book I: All chapters, including some of the more difficult exercises, either assigned or discussed in class. Chapters 1 and 2 from Book II, more as time and interest allow. Project: Either a recursive descent compiler (perhaps including Part V, the error handling routines of Chapter 6) or one using a compiler tool such as LEX/YACC.

- A full semester course (*intensive*): Book I and Chapters 1 to 10 of Book II. Project: Either of the compiler options described in *easiest* and *moderate difficulty*, or see the project outlined below for two-term sequence courses.

- Two shorter 7- to 10-week terms:

  Term I: Book I, Chapters 1 to 8, omitting Chapter 5 for a somewhat easier course. Project: Parts I–VII, omitting Part V, if desired. Do not omit Part IV even if Chapter 5 is omitted.

  Term II: Book II, Chapters 1 to 10. Project: Reimplement the compiler project (1) *using* a compiler generator or (2) *writing* a top-down parser generator as described in the addendum to Book II, Chapter 1; continue with the projects as assigned at the end of each chapter in Book II.

- A graduate course: Book II, supplemented with the Related Reading suggestions included at the end of each chapter. Project SubAda (Appendix B) if the students have no previous compiler background; PSOOL (at end of each chapter) if they have some compiler background. Both projects should use compiler tools such as LEX/YACC or create their own (top-down) parser generator.

ACKNOWLEDGMENTS

Many people and many classes have contributed to the development of this text. I would like to especially acknowledge the following people: Chris Arthur, John Casey, Michael Coomey, Robert Emmett, Larry Engholm, Enya, Gary Gray, Gary Gu, Marty Kaliski, Ellen Keohane, Kitaro, Kathy Knobe, Patti Lynch, Alok Mishra, Mat Myszewski, Kathy O'Donnell, Gary Oja, David Paist, John Potemri, Diane Ramsey, Michael Smith, Jeff Smythe, Mib Stancl, Del and Sue Webster, Jim White-head, CS 544 class, Fall 1990, CS4533 class, C Term 1991.

DESIGN OF
COMPILERS

TECHNIQUES
OF PROGRAMMING
LANGUAGE
TRANSLATION

1

Compiler Tools

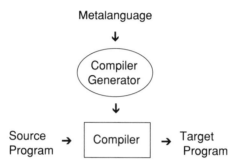

1.0 Introduction

Compiler tools aid in the generation of compilers by producing some of the phases automatically. Such tools are also called *translator writing systems, compiler compilers*, or *compiler generators*. In this book they will be referred to, most often, as *compiler generators* to emphasize that they generate a program or part of a program.

Although the picture above implies that an entire compiler can be created by a compiler generator, in fact, compiler generators cannot yet generate entire compilers automatically.

Like compilers themselves, compiler generators are frequently separated into phases. For the front end of a compiler, the phases are often termed lexical analyzer generator, syntax analyzer generator (or parser generator) and semantic analyzer generator.

As the names imply, a lexical analyzer (or scanner) generator generates a lexical analyzer (or scanner), and a syntax analyzer (or parser) generator generates a syntax analyzer (or parser).

Generator phases for the back end of compilers are still very much a research topic although work has been done on code generator generators. Figure 1 shows how a compiler generator can be parametrized. The rectangular boxes show the standard compiler phases while the ovals show the corresponding generators. The inputs to the ovals are termed *metalanguages*, which are languages that describe other languages. The front-end parts are shown grouped because often there is a single input file containing all the information needed to generate the front end of a compiler. In Figure 1, IR stands for Intermediate Representation.

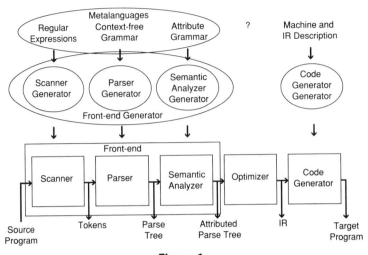

Figure 1

Scanner generators are introduced in Section 1.3 and parser generators in Section 1.4. Attribute grammars and evaluator generators are introduced in Section 1.5. For the back end, optimization and code generation will be discussed more from the point of view of automating or retargetting, and they are introduced in Sections 1.6 and 1.7. This chapter is an overview of compiler tools. Algorithms and data structures are discussed within each chapter.

1.0.1   Execution Times

There are three sets of times involved when we speak of generators: (1) generation-time, (2) compile-time, and (3) execution-time.

Generation-time is when the generator is executed: a metalanguage is input and a piece of a compiler (scanner, parser, semantic analyzer) is output.

Compile-time is when the output created at generation-time is executed: a source is input and this source is translated to another form.

Execution-time is when the code generated by the entire compiler is executed by the operating system of the machine. We won't be concerned very much with this execution-time in this text.

Some confusion arises with use of the word "execute". The generator is executed at generation-time, the compiler is executed at compile-time and the translated program is executed at execution-time.

1.1   History of Compiler Generators

By the late 1950's, computers and computer languages were proliferating. To create a compiler for N languages on M machines would require N * M programs if each were to be created separately. However, if the front-end of a compiler were to translate the source to a common intermediate language, and the back end of a compiler were to translate this intermediate language to the language of the machine, then (ideally) only N + M programs would be needed.

This was the philosophy behind UNCOL (Sammet, 1969), one of the first attempts at automating the process of compiler creation. UNCOL stood for Universal Computer-Oriented Language and was actually an intermediate language, not a compiler generator.

It proved difficult to design an intermediate language which was able to "capture" the variable aspects of different programming languages and different machines. This difficulty is still an issue in today's compiler tools. Front-end compiler generators began to appear in the early 1960's, and new generators continue to be created today.

Perhaps the best-known compiler tool is YACC, Yet Another Compiler-Compiler, written by Steve Johnson (1975). YACC runs on the UNIX operating system and is associated with another tool called LEX (Lesk and Schmidt, 1975) which generates a scanner, although it is not necessary to use a scanner generated by LEX to use YACC. The user can write his or her own scanner. LEX/YACC have been ported to other machines and operating systems.

Compiler tools whose metalanguages include attribute grammars began to appear in the late 1970's and 1980's. GAG (Kastens et al., 1982), HLP (Rai et al., 1978), VATS (Berg et al., 1984) and MUG-2 (Ganapathi et al., 1982) are based upon attribute grammar descriptions.

The PQCC (Wulf et al., 1975) project and others have undertaken the difficult task of generating the back end of a compiler.

1.2   Characteristics of Compiler Generators

A compiler tool is often designed with a particular language model in mind, and thus the tool is most suitable for generating compilers for languages similar to that model.

Like all successful software, the best compiler tools hide implementation details from the user. Since almost all tools really generate only part of the compiler, it is also very important that the tool be able to be integrated into the parts of the compiler not generated by the tool.

The largest group of compiler generators create the front-end phases of a compiler, with the back-end phases still being written by hand. Research continues into the back-end generation issues.

Four characteristics will be identified and discussed here: (1) metalanguage(s), (2) documentation, (3) functionality, and (4) outputs.

1.2.1   Metalanguage

A metalanguage describes another language or some aspect of another language. Some metalanguages for compiler parts are well known. *Regular expressions* can describe tokens, and *Backus-Naur form* (BNF) can describe the syntax of a programming language. When we add attributes and semantic functions to BNF, creating an *attribute grammar,* we can describe the semantics of a programming language, as well as the syntax.

Some metalanguages can be used to describe themselves. The term *unstratified* refers to the self-description property of a metalanguage. A good metalanguage is unstratified.

Properties of Good Metalanguages

A good metalanguage should also be easy-to-learn, easy-to-read and easy-to-use. It should be appropriate. For example, if the metalanguage is to describe tokens, it should be close to the notation for a regular expression.

A metalanguage may be "integrated", that is, have similar notations for functions throughout the different parts of the tool. For example, "=" might be used as the assignment operation for the regular expression part, the context-free part and the semantic function part. LEX and YACC use "%%" as separators between the different sections for all parts of the metalanguage.

Like programming languages themselves, the metalanguage should not contain constructs that are easily error-prone such as comments that extend over line boundaries.

A good metalanguage is difficult to define and probably a matter of taste. This section has tried to mention some properties that all metalanguages should have.

1.2.2   Documentation

The author once undertook a study of compiler tools and their characteristics (Lemone, 1987). One characteristic was seen overwhelmingly as the most important: *documentation*.

Documentation describes the tool and, as for any large or complex software package, consists of two parts: the user manual and the system documentation that describes the technical aspects of the tool. The boundary between these two can be hazy, with technical details needed to know how to use it, and using it necessary to understand the technical aspects.

Documentation for even the most widely used tools remains almost uncharted territory. The author once bought a compiler tool for her personal computer. The tool came with a manual that at first glance looked useful. But when she tried to use the manual to learn how to use the tool, she found many details missing and had several unanswered questions. A call to the company elicited the response that "they had had nothing but good comments on the manual". In fairness, the spokesperson was willing to answer the questions and, in fact, responded well to numerous phone calls.

Properties of Good Documentation

Properties of documentation for compiler tools follow many of the same rules for documentation of any software tool. Because compiler tools are complicated, on-line help is important. Most helpful, but perhaps most unlikely, is personal support from an expert on the system.

The manual should be well written and clear. A cookbook example should be included which takes the user through an application of the system. Many compiler tool manuals include a cookbook example for a so-called calculator language—often a language consisting of assignment statements with right-hand sides which are arithmetic expressions.

The cookbook example should be complete. Many cookbook examples leave "something" out, and the user is left wondering if the writers beta-tested the manual along with the software or if they hastily wrote the manual the day before the tool was released.

The documentation should be correct. Even the most innocent typographical errors can confuse a new user.

The problem of too little information versus too much information should be addressed. The documentation should include separate sections for the novice and for the more experienced user.

Most compiler tools include facilities for making changes to the generated scanner or parser (see Functionality in Section 1.2.3). At this point the user likely needs technical details about the tool. In addition, if the tool is to be maintained by a system manager, he or she will need the technical description.

Like metalanguages, good documentation is also difficult to define. With a wide range of users who have an even wider range of backgrounds, the documentation may always be seen as too elementary or too complex by the users at the ends of the spectrum.

1.2.3   Functionality

The functional characteristics of a compiler tool describe how the system works, its capabilities, and the usual software issues of extensibility, robustness, and integration.

Many generated compiler parts consist of two "pieces". The first piece is the generated table, graph or program stub (often a huge CASE statement). The second piece is a driver program that reads input and consults the table, graph or program for the next action:

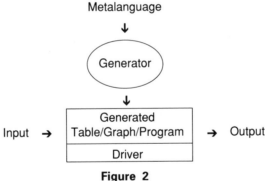

Figure 2

Some tools create tables which are then accessed by a (not generated) driver routine. Most generators now generate these tables in the form of program stubs which then are compiled and linked with the compiled driver. Although this may seem less efficient than just producing a table which is read in at the same time as the input, it allows the user to make changes, that is, to fine tune the result.

Some tools produce top-down parsers, some bottom-up. If the result is bottom-up, it may be LR(1) or LALR(1) or even something else. There are tools which produce operator precedence tables.

Some tools are parameterized. They can produce separate scanners and separate scanner/parsers as well as a scanner/parser/semantic analyzer. Some tools produce only one result—the scanner/parser/semantic analyzer or perhaps just a scanner/parser.

Most tools either generate a semantic analyzer or allow the user to write semantic routines that are executed during parsing. When the parser recognizes a construct the routine is called. Some tools allow the user to input the semantics in the form of an attribute grammar.

Properties of Good Functionality

It is harder to describe good functionality than to describe a good metalanguage or good documentation. However, some good functional characteristics are clear.

The tool should be robust; a mistake by the user shouldn't leave the user hanging with an execution error.

A tool should be efficient, both in time and in space. An inefficient tool would be one which produced the tables implemented as a single two-dimensional array. As we shall see, parse tables are sparse, and for real programming languages they are large. Data structures appropriate to sparse matrices are required.

A good tool is easily integrated with the remainder of the compiler.

A good tool has two modes of use—one for the novice that includes lots of help and prompts, and one for the sophisticated user.

1.2.4 Outputs

There are two outputs from compiler tools: (1) the tool output itself (the tables and/or program stubs) and (2) the output when the generated tool is used. We will distinguish these two by calling the first the *tool output* and the second the *resulting compiler output.*

The tool output was mentioned in Section 1.2.3. The clarity and ease of integration of the resulting outputs is important.

Many tools which generate the scanner and parser do not exactly generate the semantic analyzer. Rather, they allow the user to write routines in a high-level language, often the one generated for the program stubs of the scanner and parser. These routines are "called" when the parser makes a reduction (for bottom-up) or expands a nonterminal (for top-down).

Tools which input attribute grammars or some other notation for the semantics may generate an attribute evaluator or they may just use the semantic functions in the attribute grammar to create dependency graphs. At compile time a prewritten evaluator inputs these dependency graphs. There are other in-between techniques and they will be described in Chapter 6.

The resulting compiler output, that produced by the generated compiler itself when a source is compiled, is more difficult to describe. Some tools, notably LEX and YACC, produce no output as a default when the source program is correct. Thus, no news is good news.

This makes sense when the resulting compiler is finally integrated, debugged and put into use. However, more feedback is needed in the debugging stages, and most tools allow a range of optional outputs, sometimes added as semantic actions. The compiler project, described in the addendum to each chapter, outputs an abstract syntax tree (see the project description at the end of this chapter) as an intermediate representation.

Properties of Good Outputs

Outputs should be easy to come by. Output routines should be easy to add. For the tool output, intermediate outputs such as item sets for bottom-up parsers are helpful.

One necessary output is good error messages, that is, if the user inputs an incorrect grammar description, something more helpful than

> Incorrect grammar description

should be produced by the tool. Much research is currently devoted to this topic and we can expect future tools to be more helpful to the user.

Compile-time errors are even more difficult. To analyze this problem, realize that the compiler *generator* has to make entries into the blank portions of the generated tables or the untagged sections of CASE statements if program stubs are produced.

One technique which has met with moderate success is the use of error productions, that is, a regular expression or a BNF grammar rule is supplied which, in the generated compiler, "recognizes" an incorrect construct. The accompanying semantic action produces an appropriate error message.

1.2.5   Tool Characteristics

The preceding sections have been an attempt to provide some structure and clarity to the characteristics of compiler tools. In many cases, these characteristics are the same as those for any large software package. There are, however, characteristics and details which are particular to compiler tools.

The various features of the four characteristics are sometimes difficult to categorize. For example, error messages are part of the functionality as well as an output, and a poorly documented metalanguage may appear to be a poorly designed metalanguage (and vice versa!).

The next sections show an overview of the function of the generators. For our examples, we will use a language consisting of assignment statements whose right-hand sides consist of expressions.

1.3   Scanner Generators

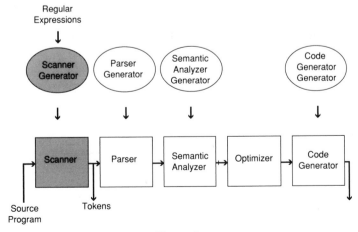

Figure 3

A scanner, or lexical analyzer, finds the elementary pieces of a program. These elements are called *tokens*.

On the generation level, the metalanguage consists of regular expressions.

These regular expressions describe tokens that the generated scanner will then be able to find when a source program is input.

Example 1 shows the regular expressions that find tokens for the components of assignment statements.

EXAMPLE 1　Regular expressions for tokens in assignment statements

```
Identifier = Letter (Letter | Digit)*
Letter = A|B|C|D|E|F|G|H|I|J|K|L|M|N|O
         |P|Q|R|S|T|U|V|W|X|Y|Z|a|b
         |c|d|e|f|g|h|i|j|k|l
         |m|n|o|p|q|r|s|t|u|v|w|x|y|z
Digit = 0|1|2|3|4|5|6|7|8|9
Operator = +|*|-|/|:=
Literal = Digit Digit*
Punctuation = ;|(|)
```

↓

Lexical
Analyzer
Generator

↓

Lexical
Analyzer

In Example 1, identifiers consist of letters and digits and begin with a letter; literals are sequences of digits; arithmetic operators are addition, subtraction, multiplication, division and assignment operators; punctuation symbols are ";" and left and right parentheses. Tokens are shown in boldface. As input to a real lexical analyzer generator, this notation would be ambiguous since the left parenthesis is used in two ways. In the definition of identifier, it is a metasymbol used for grouping, and it is an actual token in the expression for punctuation. (On the other hand, why can't a tool be designed to recognize boldface?)

Example 2 shows an input and output for the generated scanner. This example consisting of two assignment statements will be continued throughout these sections.

EXAMPLE 2   Using the generated scanner

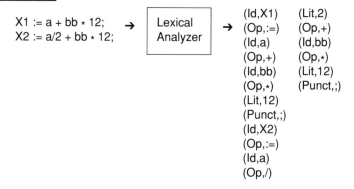

In Example 2, the two assignment statements are *tokenized*, that is, broken up into their elementary parts. Looking at the output, the reader may understand why the output is often called a token *stream*. In reality, this token stream would not be printed out except as a debugging aid when the compiler is in process of being generated (debugged).

Chapter 3 discusses the details of generating such a scanner.

1.4   Parser Generators

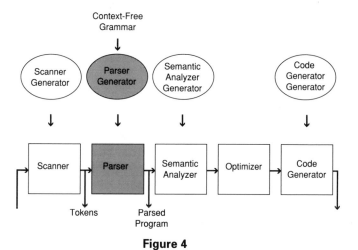

Figure 4

Figure 4 shows the input to a parser generator as a context-free grammar. Context-free grammars describe the constructs found by a parser. We will use BNF for our example. BNF is actually a notation (or yet another metalanguage) for context-free grammars. This is shown in Example 3.

EXAMPLE 3   Input to a parser generator

```
Program      →   Statements
Statements   →   Statement Statements | Statement
Statement    →   AsstStmt ;
AsstStmt     →   Identifier := Expression
Expression   →   Expression + Term | Expression - Term
                 | Term
Term         →   Term * Factor | Term / Factor
                 | Factor
Factor       →   (Expression) | Identifier | Literal
```

↓

Parser
Generator

↓

Parser

In Example 3, we see that a program consists of one or more assignment statements whose right-hand sides are arithmetic expressions. A
semicolon is used as a terminator for each assignment statement.

Example 4 shows the results when the generated parser is used. (The nonterminal
Expression has been abbreviated *Expr*.)

EXAMPLE 4   Using the generated parser

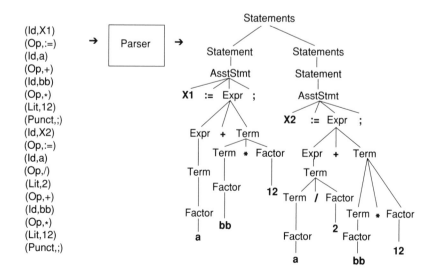

In Example 4, the tokens have been parsed, producing a parse tree. As with the generated scanner, the output is produced only during the debugging of the generated compiler pieces.

1.5   Semantic Analyzer Generators

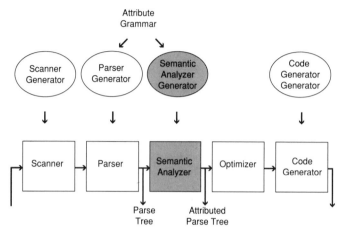

Figure 5

Figure 5 shows that the input to a semantic analyzer generator is an attribute grammar. Attribute grammars are a common specification language for semantic analysis. Because an attribute grammar is a context-free grammar with the addition of equations called semantic functions, the input is shown going to both the parser generator and the semantic analyzer generator. The context-free grammar is input to the parser generator, and the semantic functions are input to the semantic analyzer generator.

The semantic analysis phase performs many diverse tasks, rather than a single task as in scanning and parsing. Many, many variables called *attributes* are needed. In Example 5, we show only two attributes, *Use* and *Def,* which describe information about the use and definition of the variables used in the program. This information can be used to finish parsing, perhaps by warning the user that a variable has been used before it is defined. This information could also be used by the optimization phase of the compiler, perhaps by eliminating a variable that is defined, but never used. Example 5 shows an attribute grammar for the assignment statement grammar (the nonterminal *Expression* has been abbreviated *Expr*).

EXAMPLE 5   Input to a semantic analyzer generator

```
Program      → Statements        Program.Use = Statements.Use
                                  Programs.Def = Statements.Def

Statements₁  → Statement         Statement₁.Use = Statement.Use ∪
                Statements₂                       Statement₂.Use
                                  Statement₁.Def = Statement.Def ∪
                                                   Statements₂.Def:

Statements   → Statement         Statements.Use = Statement.Use

                                  Statements.Def = Statement.Def

Statement    → AsstStmt          Statement.Use = Asst.Use
                                  Statement.Def = Asst.Def

AsstStmt     → Identifier :=      AsstStmt.Def = {LexVal(Identifier)}
                Expr              AsstStmt.Use = {Expr.Use}


Expr₁        → Expr₂ + Term       Expr₁.Use = Expr₂.Use ∪ Term.Use
              | Expr₂ - Term      Expr₁.Use = Expr₂.Use ∪ Term.Use
              | Term              Expr₁.Use = Term.Use

Term₁        → Term₂ * Factor     Term₁.Use = Term₂.Use ∪ Factor.Use
              | Term₂ /           Term₁.Use = Term₂.Use ∪ Factor.Use
                Factor
              | Factor            Term₁.Use = Factor.Use

Factor       → ( Expr)            Factor.Use = Expr.Use
              | Identifier        Factor.Use = {LexVal(Identifier)}
              |Literal            Literal.Use = { }
```

↓

(Semantic
Analyzer
Generator)

↓

Semantic
Analyzer

Example 5 shows the input of an attribute grammar to the semantic analyzer genera.or. The two attributes, *Use* and *Def,* are associated with various nonterminals in the grammar. At parse time the nodes will be labeled with these (unevaluated) attributes, and at semantic analysis time the values of these attributes will be evaluated by propagating information up the parse tree. Example 6 shows the results produced by the generated semantic analyzer.

1.6   Optimization and Optimizer Generators

EXAMPLE 6   Using the generated semantic analyzer

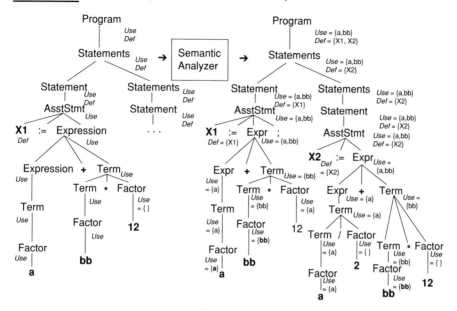

Example 6 shows that the values have been computed for the attributes *Use* and *Def*. The input to the semantic evaluator is an unattributed parse tree, so the parser has done something more than that shown in Section 1.4. The entire parse tree input is not shown because of lack of space (see Exercise 3). The values of *Use* and *Def* at the top of the tree (the node program) might be used to issue the messages:

```
X1,X2 defined but not used
a,bb used but not defined
```

if this were an entire program.

The line between semantic analysis and optimization is fuzzy. If the information about the use and definition of variables from Section 1.5 were used to allocate values to registers, then we might term the process optimization. Also, code generation may make optimizations, both before and after code is selected. Optimizations on the generated code are called *peephole* optimizations.

The optimization process changes the intermediate representation so that the code ultimately generated executes faster or takes up less space.

Optimization can calculate more attribute values, or it can change the tree itself, or it may even change the intermediate representation to a graph and make changes to the graph.

Chapters 6 to 8 discuss these various options. We will defer examples until those sections.

1.7   Code Generation and Code Generator Generators

A code generator generator inputs a description of the machine and intermediate representation and outputs a code generator. A code generator outputs object code. Here, we will settle for assembly language. There are other steps which are taken toward automating the code generation process that are something less than a code generator generator.

A first step toward automating the code generation process, and good programming style as well, is to separate the code generation algorithm from the machine code itself. This allows tables of (IR,Code) couples to be created and used and perhaps changed to be ported to another machine.

Example 7 shows a code generator that might be termed *retargetable*. Input to the code generator (not a code generator-generator) is a description of a subtree of the intermediate representation to be matched and code to be output based upon the match. If there were a code generator generator, its input would include a description of the machine.

EXAMPLE 7   Retargetable code generation

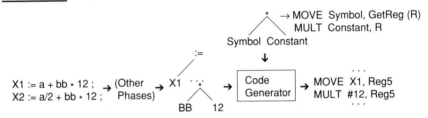

In Example 7, at code generator *generation* time, tables are created which describe abstract syntax tree patterns to be matched (at code generation time) and the code to be generated. Thus, the pattern for an abstract syntax (sub)tree node whose root is a * *operator* and whose children are a *symbol* and a *constant* is stored together with the code that gets the next available register and emits a move instruction and a multiply instruction. At code generation time, when an abstract syntax tree that matches this is input, the code is output. This is called *retargetable* since the tables can be easily changed to output code for another machine.

1.8   Summary

This chapter has introduced the phases of a compiler. Front-end phases are lexical analysis and syntax analysis, while back-end phases are optimization and code generation. Semantic analysis tends to overlap both the front end, which focuses on the language being *analyzed,* and back-end phases which focus on the code being *synthesized.*

The remainder of this book presents algorithms and data structures for performing and/or generating these compiler phases. Where possible, mainly for the front end, we focus on automating the compiling process. Where automation is more difficult, mainly in the back end, we focus on techniques for efficient processing.

Compilers are an interesting, integrated computer science topic, encompassing concepts from data structures, algorithms, computability, computer architecture and software engineering, to name a few. In addition, topics in compiler design continue to evolve: new architectures (see Chapter 12) require new techniques; the automation process continues to be researched and developed; error processing techniques continue to improve.

Building the right tools and good design produce good compilers.

1.9   Related Reading

Aho, A. V. 1980. Translator Writing Systems: Where Do They Now Stand?, *IEEE Computer*, August: 9–13.

Berg, A. et al. 1984. *VATS—The Visible Attributed Translation System*, Technical Report 84–19, Saskatoon: Department of Computational Science, University of Saskatchewan.

Dobler, H. and K. Pirklbauer. 1990. Coco-2, A New Compiler Compiler, *SIGPLAN Notices*, 25(5):82–90.

Ganapathi, M. J., J. L. Hennessy, and C. N. Fischer. 1982. Retargetable Compiler Code Generation, *Computing Surveys*, 14(4):573–592.

Ganzinger, H. et al. 1977. Automatic Generation of Optimizing Multipass Compilers, in *Information Processing 77*, Amsterdam: North-Holland.

Hammer, (ed). 1989. *Compiler Compilers and High Speed Compilation*, #371, Lecture Notes in Computer Science, New York: Springer-Verlag.

Harapriyan, H. K., Y. N. Srikant, and P. Shankar. 1988. A Compiler Writing System Based on Affix Grammars, *Computer Languages*, 13(1).

Johnson, S. C. 1975. *Yet Another Compiler Compiler*, C. S. Technical Report #32, Murray Hill, NJ: Bell Telephone Laboratories.

Kastens, U., B. Hott, and E. Zimmerman. 1982. *GAG: A Practical Compiler Generator*, Lecture Notes in Computer Science, 141, Berlin: Springer-Verlag.

Lemone, K. A. 1987. *A Language Processing Laboratory*, in Proceedings of the 1987 ACM/CSE Conference, St. Louis.

Lesk, M. E. and E. Schmidt. 1975. A Lexical Analyzer Generator, in *UNIX Programmer's Manual 2*, Murray Hill, NJ: AT&T Bell Laboratories.

Raiha, K. J., M. Saarinen, E. Soisanion-Soininen, and M. Tienari. 1978. *The Compiler Writing System HLP*, Report A-1978-2, Dept. of Computer Science, Univ. of Helsinki, Finland.

Sammet, J. E. 1969. *Programming Languages: History and Fundamentals*, Englewood Cliffs, NJ: Prentice-Hall.

Shepard, J. C. 1991. Why a Two Pass Front End?, *SIGPLAN Notices*, 26(3):88–94.

Wulf, W. A., R. K. Johnson, C. B. Wienstock, S. O. Hobbs, and G. M. Geschke. 1975. *The Design of an Optimizing Compiler*, Amsterdam: Elsevier-North Holland.

Background Reading

Aho, A. V., R. Sethi, and J. D. Ullman. 1985. *Compilers: Principles, Techniques, Tools*, Reading, MA: Addison-Wesley.

Fischer, C. N. and R. J. LeBlanc, Jr. 1988. *Crafting a Compiler*, Menlo Park, CA: Benjamin/Cummings.

Lemone, K. A. 1992. *Fundamentals of Compilers*, Boca Raton, FL: CRC Press.

EXERCISES

1. What characteristics could be added to those listed in Section 1.2 for (a) good metalanguage design, (b) good documentation, (c) good functionality, and (d) good outputs?

2. Consider a language of copy statements. Both the left-hand side and the right-hand side contain identifiers. The following is a "program" in this language:

   ```
   Max := A;
   This := That;
   ```

   (a) Show the input to a lexical analyzer generator.
   (b) Show the output from the resulting lexical analyzer.
   (c) Show the input to a parser generator.
   (d) Show the output from the resulting parser.

3. Finish the parse tree and corroborate the attribute values for the parse tree of Example 6.

4. What are three possible functions of the optimization process?

5. Create all the templates as in Example 7 to output code for the two assignment statements.

6. List and show an example of the metalanguages for each part of the compiler.

7. Modify the regular expression for identifier to include "$" and "_" after the leading letter.

8. Using the set of productions shown in Example 3, show that

   ```
   y := z + 1 - x * 5
   ```

   is a statement.

9. Discuss the pros and cons of few versus many classes for tokens.

Project

This project can easily take an entire term or semester. If the project described in the rest of this book is to be done, then this project needs to be limited to a week or two (at most!).

Research and compare several compiler tools, comparing them for the four characteristics: documentation, metalanguage, functionality, and outputs.

When writing up your results, take into account any other pertinent information: your background, technical support, etc.

Use the grammar for assignment statements found in the chapter as the common example.

2

Language Design

2.0 Introduction

Throughout this text, we focus on language design issues from an implementation point of view. Certainly, the compiler implementation influences the language design. The programming language Ada was designed over a period of years (DOD, 1977, 1978, 1980, 1983) with experienced compiler designers as key members of the design team. Because of this, certain features such as static binding (the specification of attributes of all types before execution time) became part of the language design.

Other languages such as SmallTalk (BYTE, 1981; Goldberg and Robson, 1983) were designed to aid the problem solving process. Efficient implementations came later.

Designing a language and designing its implementation go hand in hand. Efficient compilers have made (Ada) or broken (early versions of PL/I) a language.

2.0.1 Language Design Issues

Various issues have been identified for designing a programming language. Donahue (1990) mentions four aspects. The first is the *mathematical aspect* which dictates that the language be elegant, but simple to describe mathematically. Lisp-like languages are an example of languages for which this aspect is particularly noticeable.

Other ways to describe this aspect are to say that the language should have an inherent simplicity and be easy to learn, expressive and orthogonal. Expressiveness is the power of the language to solve problems. Orthogonality requires combinations of legal constructs to be themselves legal constructs. Thus, if a user type of stack is created, and the language allows arrays, an array of stacks would also be allowed. This feature is somewhat related to polymorphism, described below.

Included in the mathematical aspect is the ability of the language's syntax and semantics to be described accurately and precisely.

The second aspect is the cognitive and social aspect, the so-called programmer's language. The programming language C is an example of a language with high programmer visibility. It should be easy to read and write programs in the language. Most people would agree that it is easy, with programming maturity, to write programs in C, but reading them is more difficult. Modula-3 programs are both easy to read and easy to write.

The third aspect, an important one, is its implementation: How many person-months does it take to construct the compiler? How large is it? How fast is it?

Niklaus Wirth (1976), the designer of Pascal, states that a "programming language is as good as its compiler".

The fourth aspect is a marketing aspect. C++, an object-oriented version of C, is aggressively marketed and this has affected its use.

Others (Ghezzi and Jazayeri, 1987) have emphasized the relationship between programming language design and software design methodology. At the present state-of-the-art, this would lead us to the design of a programming language which supports information hiding and data abstraction.

In this chapter, we will consider a language design which follows the object-oriented programming paradigm. We will borrow freely from other languages; the control structures will be very Pascal-like. We will consider features such as persistence and inheritance; then we will devise some ways to describe them syntactically.

2.0.2   Language Design as an Example of the Software Design Process

A language is, itself, a software system or part of a software system. The five standard phases of the software development process can provide a structure in which to develop a language (and then we can apply these phases all over again to its compiler!).

The first phase is *requirements analysis and specification*. The language we will design, PSOOL, will meet requirements and specifications from the object-oriented paradigm.

The second phase is *software design and specification*. We can apply this to language design by specifying a syntax and a semantics for PSOOL.

The third phase, *implementation,* is the compiler and, as mentioned above, is a software system in its own right.

The fourth phase, *certification*, or validation checks that the implementation, the compiler, satisfies the syntactic and semantic description.

The fifth phase, *maintenance*, is somewhat different for language design since a language shouldn't really change until a new version is needed. However, languages such as Modula were followed by Modula-2 and then by Modula-3, so enhancements do take place. FORTRAN has steadily evolved over the years.

Exercise 1 asks the reader to describe the five phases for the compiler itself.

The next section describes object-oriented languages and the features which will be included in the project whose parts are described at the end of each chapter. If the alternate project (SubAda) described in Appendix B (or an extensive version of the project described at the end of Chapter 1) is to be done, then the remaining sections of this chapter may be read briefly or skipped.

2.1   Concepts of Object-Oriented Languages

Object-oriented concepts evolved from the *encapsulation* and *information hiding* of abstract data types. Briefly, encapsulation allows operations to be defined for a type. The *push* and *pop* operations for a *stack* object are a classic example. Information hiding prevents the user of these operations and objects from seeing how these operations and objects are implemented. The stack may be implemented as a linear list, as an array or as some other data structure; the *push* and *pop* operations are, similarly, implemented in a way which is invisible to the user. The user merely creates a stack object and uses the push and pop operations.

Object-oriented languages include more features than just encapsulation and information hiding. These features include *messages, methods, inheritance, overloading, polymorphism, persistence* and *late-binding* (Cox, 1986; Schriver and Wegner, 1988).

In this chapter, we adopt the object-oriented definitions from Wegner (1987) and Nelson (1991). Thus, an object-oriented language supports objects which, themselves, belong to classes. The classes are hierarchically connected by an inheritance mechanism. In addition, we consider persistence, polymorphism and late-binding.

2.1.1   Objects, Classes and Data Abstraction

Objects are dynamic data on which dynamic actions are performed and which have a state. A class is a static grouping to which similar objects belong and under whose auspices new objects may be created. The data are described by variables and behavior is characterized by permitted operations. The *Stack* might be declared as a class and *MyStack* as one of the objects in this class.

Data abstraction hides the internal representation of the data and the implementation of the operations. The user specifies *what* operation is to be performed, not *how* the operation is to be performed.

2.1.2   Messages and Methods

Data abstraction prevents an object's data from being directly manipulated. To perform an operation on an object, a message is sent. The message contains a selector which tells the object what to do. The message may also contain parameters to aid in the operation or through which the object may return values. For example, the message *MyStack: Push (3)* might send a message to the object *MyStack* telling it to push the integer 3 onto *MyStack*.

A class groups actions (called methods) and variables (called instance variables). When an object of a particular class receives a message to perform an action, it finds the method(s) corresponding to the message selector and performs the action. Corresponding to the selector *Push* for the message *MyStack: Push (3)* is a method or methods known to the *Stack* class (which might also be called *Push*) which accomplishes the operation. How this happens is unknown to the procedure which sent the message.

In the bank example in Section 2.4, a message is sent to an object in the *Savings Account* class telling it to generate an account number for a new *SavingsAccount*. *GenerateAccountNumber* is the selector in the message. The sender of the message does not know how this number is generated. The object *SavingsAccount* invokes its method, *GenerateAccountNumber,* to generate the account number.

Two types of variables are allowed in our model—class variables whose values vary for each object instance of that class and shared variables whose values are common and accessible to all object instances of a class.

2.1.3   Subclasses, Superclasses and Inheritance

Reusability of software is enhanced via inheritance, a technique for defining new classes, called subclasses, in terms of existing classes. These new classes are defined by describing how they are similar to and how they differ from their preexisting superclasses. They may share the same or similar memory layout and respond to messages with the same or slightly altered methods.

A subclass is said to inherit characteristics of its superclass, enabling the creation of classes which are very similar to other classes, thus saving a lot of "programmer" time. Multiple inheritance allows a class to inherit from more than one superclass. Altering a method or an instance variable from that of a superclass is referred to as *specialization*. In our model, inheritance of data and methods is stated explicitly. This does not require the programmer to write (much) more code and is worth the tradeoff in safety.

In the bank example, the *BankAccount* class has two subclasses, *CheckingAccount* and *SavingsAccount*. These subclasses inherit many, but not all, of the methods of *BankAccount*. A class called *NOWAccount* is defined as an example of multiple inheritance since it is a subclass of both *CheckingAccount* and *SavingsAccount* and inherits from both. For *NOWAccount,* one of the inherited methods, *GetInterestRate*, is specialized by appending a method, *CheckForMinimumBalance*, to the beginning.

2.1.4   Overloading and Polymorphism

Overloading allows an operator to operate on more than one data type. For example, virtually all languages allow "+" to operate on both integer and real type data. Polymorphism extends this capability to allow procedures to operate on different types and functions to return values of different types on different calls (Harland, 1984). For example, a procedure *Sort* would be polymorphic if it could be used as the selector in a message to both an integer array object and a character array object. The objects themselves would invoke methods corresponding to the selector to perform the appropriate actions. In the bank example in Section 2.4.2, for (simple) polymorphism, *GetInterestRate* is the selector in a message to both a *SavingsAccount* object and a *NOWAccount* object.

2.1.5   Late Binding

Binding is the attachment of a name to a value in a program. Binding-time refers to when this association is made. Thus a compile-time binding ties a name to a value before the program even begins to execute.

Here, we regard binding as the process whereby object operations and operands are combined. Early binding combines them at compile time (static binding) or even before, during program writing time and is implemented with case statements (or their equivalent) which must be changed if a new data type is to be included for the operation.

Late binding combines operations and operands as late as when the program is running (dynamic binding). Messages often require dynamic binding—in our example, the message to tell an account to add interest to the balance involves dynamic binding since the type of account is not known at compile time (see Late-Binding example in Section 2.4).

2.1.6   Persistence

Persistence is a property of object-oriented systems which allows, or requires, objects to exist from one execution of a program to another. Database techniques are often involved in persistent systems.

Persistence is related to binding in the sense that newly created objects and previously created objects need to be bound to some storage mechanism so that they may be reused.

2.1.7   PSOOL — A Pseudo Object-Oriented Language

Now that we have specified some object-oriented concepts, we are ready to design our language. It may not be clear which of the concepts are described via syntax, which via semantics or both. In the next section, we will see that classes, messages, methods, subclasses, superclasses, and inheritance all have a syntactic element as well as a semantic element while persistence, polymorphism and late binding are purely semantic.

2.2   PSOOL Syntax

In this section, we develop a BNF grammar to describe PSOOL.

2.2.1   Algorithmic vs. Functional vs. Logic vs. . . .

There are many categories of programming languages. Languages such as Pascal, Ada and C are algorithmic. Lisp, Scheme and others are functional in notation. Prolog's syntax, as well as its semantics, is based on the notation of predicate logic.

We will make the decision that our notation will be algorithmic. Then, we will freely borrow control constructs for loops and conditionals from these languages. Although the syntax will be somewhat different, we will be, in some sense, reinventing SmallTalk^{TM}, the system from which these concepts all came. SmallTalk^{TM}, however, is a functional language.

2.2.2   BNF for PSOOL

The extended BNF notation includes brackets, [ ], and braces, { }. Brackets indicate optional items; braces indicate 0 or more occurrences of the contents, and { }$^+$ indicates 1 or more occurrences of the contents.

The notation __Name indicates any category which ends in "Name": *Method-Name*. Tokens are boldfaced or italicized. Non-bolded parentheses are used as metasymbols for grouping; when parentheses, (and), are used as tokens, they are bolded.

The start symbol for PSOOL is Program. A PSOOL program (Figure 1) consists of one or more class descriptions followed by one or more actions:

```
1. Program →{ClassDescription}+ {Action}+

2. ClassDescription →
   Class        ClassName ;
   SuperClass
        (SuperClassNames ; | None ; )
   InstanceVariables
     ({Inherit        InheritClassNames
     From ClassName ; }+  |    Inherit None ; )
     Introduce InstanceVariableDeclarations
        | None ; )
```

Figure 1   BNF for PSOOL

SharedVariables
  ({**Inherit** SharedVarNames}
  From ClassName ;}$^+$ | **Inherit None** ;)
  Introduce SharedVariableDeclarations
        | **None** ;)
  Methods (Methods| **None**) ;
  EndClass ClassName ;

3. Methods   →
      ({**Inherit**   InheritMethodNames
          From ClassName ;}$^+$ | **Inherit None** ;)
      Introduce (IntroMethodNames
          | **None**) ;
      ({({**Specialize** SpecializeMethodName
      With MethodName **Before** ;}$^+$
      |{**Specialize** SpecializeMethodName
      With MethodName **After** ;}$^+$)}$^+$
          | **SpecializeNone** ;)
      Definitions (Definitions
          | **None**) ;

4. Definitions →
      {**Method** MethodName ;
          | MethodName
          (ParameterNames) ;
      LocalNames
          LocalNames ; | **None** ;
      BeginMethod
          SequenceOfStatements
      EndMethod MethodName}$^+$

5. Action → **Action** ActionName ;
                LocalNames LocalVariableDeclarations
                        | **None** ;
            BeginAction
                SequenceOfStatements
            EndAction ActionName ;

6 _VariableDeclarations →
        {Names : TypeDefinition [:= Expression]} ;

7. TypeDefinition → StandardType | ClassName

8. StandardType → Integer | Float | Char | String | Boolean

9. SequenceOfStatements → {Statement ; }$^+$

10. Statement → Assignment
                    | Selection
                    | Loop

Figure 1 (continued)

| Instantiation
| Message
| **Return** (Expression)
| **Read** (Names)
| **Write** (Expression)

11. Assignment → Name := Expression

12. Selection → **IF** Expression **THEN**
           SequenceOfStatements
           { **ELSIF** Expression **THEN**
           SequenceOfStatements }
           [**ELSE**
           SequenceOfStatements]
         ENDIF

13. Loop → [IterationScheme] LOOP SequenceOf-
           Statements
       ENDLOOP

13.25. IterationScheme → **WHILE** *Boolean*Expression
           | **For** *Identifier* in DiscreteRange

13.5. DiscreteRange → SimpleExpression..SimpleEx-
           pression

14. Instantiation → Name := **New** (ClassName[,*Parame-*
           *ter*Names])
           | Name := **Get** (ClassName[,*Para-*
           *meter*Names])

15. Message → *Object*Name : Selector [**(** *Parameter-*
           Names **)**]

16. Selector → *Method*Name

17. Expression → Relation
           | Expression **AND** Relation
           | Expression **OR** Relation
           | Expression **XOR** Relation

18. Relation → SimpleExpression
           | SimpleExpression RelationalOperator
               SimpleExpression

19. SimpleExpression → Term { AddingOperator Term }

20. Term → Factor { MultiplyingOperator Factor }

21. Factor → Primary | **NOT** Primary | [UnaryOperator]
           Primary

22. Primary → Name | NumericLiteral | (Expression)
           | Message

Figure 1 (continued)

```
23.  __Names  →  __Name [ : Type ] ;
                  | __Names , Name [ : Type ] ;
24.  __Name  →  SimpleName | Name [(ExpressionList)]
25. ExpressionList  →  Expression
                          | Expressionlist , Expression
26. SimpleName  →  Identifier
27. NumericLiteral  →  Integer
28. AddingOperator = + | -
29. MultiplyingOperator = * | / | mod
30. RelationalOperator = = | <> | > | < | >= | <=
```
Figure 1 (continued)

Note that it is left to the particular implementation to decide on the definition of legal identifiers or types. The BNF in Figure 1 is the author's creation from the ideas of the previous sections. Many variations of this syntax are possible, and the reader is invited to add his or her own touches. Some suggestions are made in the exercises.

2.3   PSOOL Semantics

Describing programming language semantics has proved elusive. Notations which are easy to understand tend not to be precise, and notations which are precise tend to be very difficult to understand.

Historically, programming language semantics has been described by three different methods: *operational* semantics, *axiomatic* semantics and *denotational* semantics. These are successively more formal, difficult to understand, and precise.

Formal semantic discussions are outside the range of this book, but we include several references in the Related Reading at the end of the chapter.

2.3.1   Operational Semantics

The operational semantics of a programming language describes the language as its behavior when a program in the language executes. Often, this is in terms of an abstract computer rather than a specific computer.

2.3.2   Axiomatic Semantics

The axiomatic semantics of a programming language is that used in program proving. For each statement there is a precondition that describes the possibilities which may exist before a statement is executed. A postcondition describes the possibilities after the statement executes given a particular precondition.

2.3.3   Denotational Semantics

Denotational semantics describes programming languages mathematically. The atomic elements are described in terms of their properties and then other elements are described in terms of the constituent elements.

2.3.4 "Implementational" Semantics

For PSOOL, we will use a somewhat operational approach, defining the meaning informally using the object-oriented definitions in Section 2.1. The implementation of these constructs will be facilitated using attribute grammars. This is best seen by showing a PSOOL application.

2.4 A PSOOL Application

We will create a PSOOL program to implement a banking system. To understand the meaning of Actions, we will write several actions which will operate on an abstract notion of a *BankAccount*. A *BankAccount* may be a *SavingsAccount*, a *CheckingAccount*, and a combination account called a NOW account. The specific actions will illustrate the object-oriented concepts from Section 2.1. The implementation of the classes will be shown after the example of their use, thus reinforcing the idea of information hiding.

2.4.1 Action Showing Inheritance, Object Instantiation and Messaging

The following example creates a *SavingsAccount*.

```
Action  CreateNewSavingsAccount ;
  LocalNames
        CompoundInterestRate : Integer := 6 ;
{ThisAccount used for instantiation of savings
account object}
        ThisAccount : SavingsAccount ;
{IO used for instantiation of a utilities object}
        IO : Utilities ;
BeginAction {CreateNewSavingsAccount}
{Instantiate a savings account object}
  ThisAccount := New(SavingsAccount) ;
{Instantiate a Utilities object }
  IO := New(Utilities);
  { Send messages to object utilities and to object
    savings account to set fields }
  IO : PutPrompt ("Owner?") ;
  IO : Input (Owner) ;
  ThisAccount : SetOwner(Owner) ;
  IO : PutPrompt ("Address?") ;
  IO : Input (Address) ;
  ThisAccount: SetAddress (Address) ;
  IO : PutPrompt ("PhoneNumber?") ;
  IO : Input (PhoneNumber) ;
  ThisAccount :
        SetPhoneNumber(PhoneNumber) ;
  ThisAccount : GenerateAccountNumber ;
  IO : PutPrompt ("InitialDeposit") ;
  IO : Input (InitialDeposit) ;
```

```
    ThisAccount : DepositFunds (InitialDeposit) ;
    ThisAccount : AddInterestToBalance ;

EndAction CreateNewSavingsAccount ;
```

Here, the object *SavingsAccount* is created and messages are sent to it. The names of the corresponding methods will be found in the data declaration for a *Savings Account* .

2.4.2 Polymorphism

The action in this section illustrates polymorphism by sending a message with the same selector (*AddInterestToBalance*) to two different objects.

```
Action AddInterest ;
{Example shows simple polymorphism—can be resolved
  at compile time}
Local Names
{Account1 used for instantiation of a NOWAccount
  object}
Account1 : NOWAccount ;
{Account2 used for instantiation of a Savings
  Account object}
Account2 : SavingsAccount ;
{IO used for instantiation of a Utilities object}
  IO : Utilities ;
AccountName:String ;
BeginAction {AddInterest}
  IO := NEW(Utilities) ;
  IO : Input(AccountName) ;
  Account1 := GET(Account1,AccountName) ;
{Presumably, AccountName has 2 different accounts}
  Account2 := GET(Account2,AccountName) ;
  Account1 : AddInterestToBalance ;
  Account2 : AddInterestToBalance ;

EndAction AddInterest ;
```

2.4.3 Late-Binding

Dynamic binding is a philosophy basic to many object-oriented programming environments; yet, it is often admitted that dynamic binding is a flexibility that is paid for in terms of efficiency. The solution may be to do as much bookkeeping at compile time as possible to facilitate dynamic binding. Below is an example which shows a message that is sent to an object whose identity is not known until run-time (since the object type itself is an input value):

```
Action AddInterest ;

{Example shows late-binding}

Local Names
{Used for instantiation of an account object}
```

```
Account : BankAccount ;
AccountType : ClassName ;
AccountName : String ;
Deposit : Real ;
{Used for instantiation of a Utilities object}
IO : Utilities ;
```

BeginAction {AddInterest}

```
IO := NEW(Utilities) ;
IO : Input(AccountType) ;
IO : Input(AccountName) ;
IO : Input(Deposit) ;
Account := NEW(AccountType) ;
Account : DepositFunds(Deposit) ;
Account : AddInterestToBalance ;
```

EndAction AddInterest ;

Here, the specific object, whether it be a *SavingsAccount*, a *CheckingAccount* or a *NOWAccount* is not known until run-time. The next four examples show class declarations using PSOOL syntax.

2.4.4 Class Descriptions

We will define a *Utilities* Class which will isolate the I/O for our example.

```
Class Utilities ;
  SuperClass    None ;
  InstanceVariables ;
    Inherit    None ;
    Introduce    None ;
  SharedVariables
    Inherit    None ;
    Introduce    None ;
  Methods
    Inherit    None ;
    Introduce
      Input,
      PutPrompt ;
    Specialize None ;
  Definitions
    Method Input (Info) ;
      LocalNames None ;
      BeginMethod  {Input}
        Read(Info) ;
      EndMethod Input ;
    Method PutPrompt (Info) ;
      LocalNames None ;
      BeginMethod {PutPrompt}
        Write (Info) ;
```

```
        EndMethod PutPrompt ;
    EndClass Utilities ;
```

The next class description is for a *BankAccount*. Like the *Utilities* Class, it has no superclass. We will see, however, that this class is a superclass of other classes.

```
Class    BankAccount ;
  SuperClass      None ;
  InstanceVariables
    Inherit    None ;
    Introduce
      Owner,
      Address,
      PhoneNumber : String ;
      AccountNumber : Integer ;
      Balance : Real ;
  SharedVariables
    Inherit None ;
    Introduce
      HighInterestRate : real := 0.07 ;
      LowInterestRate : real := 0.045 ;
      NextAccountNumber : real := 0 ;
  Methods
    Inherit    None ;
    Introduce
      GetInterestRate,
      DepositFunds,
      SetOwner,
      SetAddress,
      SetPhoneNumber,
      GenerateAccountNumber ;
    Specialize    None ;
  Definitions
    Method GetInterestRate ;
      LocalNames None ;
      BeginMethod {GetInterestRate}
      If (Balance > 10000) Then
      Return (HighInterestRate) ;
      Else
        Return (LowInterestRate) ;
      EndIf ;
    EndMethod GetInterestRate ;
    Method DepositFunds
        (AmountDeposited) ;
      LocalNames None ;
      BeginMethod {Deposit Funds}
        Balance := Balance + AmountDeposited ;
      EndMethod DepositFunds ;
    Method SetOwner (Name) ;
```

```
          LocalNames None ;
          BeginMethod {SetOwner}
            Owner := Name ;
      EndMethod SetOwner ;
      Method SetAddress(Name) ;
        LocalNames None ;
        BeginMethod {SetAddress}
          Address := Name ;
      EndMethod SetAddress ;
      Method SetPhoneNumber (Number) ;
        LocalNames None ;
        BeginMethod {SetPhoneNumber}
          PhoneNumber := Number ;
      EndMethod SetPhoneNumber ;
      Method GenerateAccountNumber ;
        LocalNames None ;
        BeginMethod
          {GenerateAccountNumber}
          NextAccountNumber := NextAccountNumber + 1 ;
          AccountNumber := NextAccountNumber ;
      EndMethod GenerateAccountNumber ;

    EndClass BankAccount ;
```

2.4.5 Subclasses

The next class is a *SavingsAccount* class which is a subclass of *BankAccount* and inherits some methods from it.

```
    Class    SavingsAccount ;
      SuperClass
        BankAccount ;
      InstanceVariables
        Inherit
          Owner,
          Address,
          PhoneNumber,
          AccountNumber,
          Balance
        From BankAccount ;
        Introduce None ;
      SharedVariables
        Inherit
          HighInterestRate := 0.07 ;
          LowInterestRate := 0.045 ;
          NextAccountNumber := 0 ;
        Introduce None ;
      Methods
        Inherit
```

```
              GetInterestRate,
              DepositFunds,
              SetOwner,
              SetAddress,
              SetPhoneNumber,
              GenerateAccountNumber
        From BankAccount ;
        Inherit
           Input,
           PutPrompt
        From Utilities ;
        Introduce WithdrawFunds,
           AddInterestToBalance ;
        Specialize  None ;
     Definitions
        Method WithdrawFunds (AmountRequested) ;
        LocalNames IO ;
        BeginMethod {WithdrawFunds}
        If (AmountRequested >
           Balance) Then
        IO := New(Utilities) ;
        IO: PutPrompt ("Amount requested higher than
                        balance") ;
        Else Balance := Balance—AmountRequested ;
        EndIf ;
     EndMethod WithdrawFunds ;
     Method AddInterestToBalance ;
     LocalNames InterestRate ;
     BeginMethod {AddInterestToBalance}
     InterestRate := self : GetInterestRate ;
        Balance := Balance + Balance * InterestRate ;
     EndMethod AddInterestToBalance ;
   EndClass  SavingsAccount ;
```

The next class description, *CheckingAccount*, is also a subclass of a *BankAccount*.

```
   Class    CheckingAccount ;
     SuperClass    BankAccount ;
     InstanceVariables
        Inherit
           Owner,
           Address,
           PhoneNumber,
           AccountNumber
           Balance
        From BankAccount ;
     Introduce
        JointAccount,
        SecondAccountHolder ;
```

```
      SharedVariables
         Inherit
            HighInterestRate := 0.07 ;
            LowInterestRate := 0.045 ;
            NextAccountNumber:= 0 :
         From BankAccount
         Introduce
            BounceFee : Real := 12.50 ;
      Methods
         Inherit
            DepositFunds,
            {GetInterestRate removed}
            SetOwner,
            SetAddress,
            SetPhoneNumber,
            GenerateAccountNumber,
         From BankAccount ;
         Introduce
            ClearCheck ;
         Specialize     None ;
         Definitions
         Method
            ClearCheck(CheckAmount) ;
         LocalNames None ;
         BeginMethod {ClearCheck}
            If (CheckAmount >
               Balance) Then
            New(Utilities) ;
               IO : PutPrompt ("Amount requested higher
                               than balance") ;
            Balance := Balance—BounceFee ;
            Else Balance := Balance—CheckAmount ;
            EndIf ;
         EndMethod ClearCheck ;
   EndClass CheckingAccount ;
```

2.4.6 Multiple Inheritance

The next class is a subclass of both *SavingsAccount* and *CheckingAccount*, inheriting from both. Although the method *GetInterestRate* is inherited from *SavingsAccount*, it is specialized by adding some code to the beginning.

```
      Class    NOWAccount ;
         SuperClass
            SavingsAccount,
            CheckingAccount ;
         InstanceVariables
            Inherit
               Owner,
```

```
            Address,
            PhoneNumber,
            Balance,
            AccountNumber
            JointAccount,
            SecondAccountHolder
        From CheckingAccount ;
        Introduce None ;
    SharedVariables
        Inherit
            HighInterestRate := 0.07 ;
            LowInterestRate := 0.045 ;
            NextAccountNumber:= 0 ;
        Introduce None ;
    Methods
        Inherit
            GetInterestRate,
            DepositFunds,
            SetOwner,
            SetAddress,
            SetPhoneNumber,
            GenerateAccountNumber,
            WithdrawFunds,
            AddInterestToBalance
        From Savings Account ;
        Inherit
            ClearCheck
        From  CheckingAccount ;
        Introduce  None ;
        Specialize
            GetInterestRate
        With CheckForMinimumBalance
        Before ;
    Definitions
        Method
            CheckForMinimumBalance
            LocalNames None ;
            BeginMethod
            {CheckForMinimumBalance }
            If (Balance < 1000) Then
                Return (0) ;
            EndIf ;
        EndMethod CheckForMinimumBalance ;
    EndClass NOWAccount ;
```

2.5   Implementing PSOOL

PSOOL may be implemented using LEX and YACC or any other compiler tool to create the scanner (see Chapter 3) and parser (see Chapters 4 and 5). We will use attributes and attribute grammars to implement semantics (see Chapter 6). The next section shows parse trees for the class declarations. (The reader may wish to go straight to symbol table creation for these.)

2.5.1   The Parse Trees

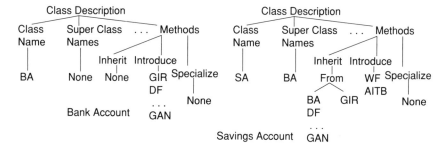

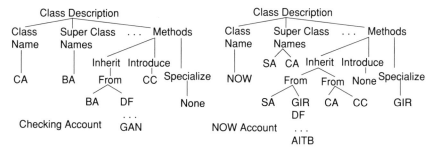

Figure 2 Parse Trees

For the four classes of interest here, *BankAccount* (*BA*), *SavingsAccount* (*SA*), *CheckingAccount* (*CA*) and *NOWAccount* (*NOW*), trees are shown above. Nodes that are not of interest here (e.g., Shared Variables) are not shown for simplicity. Method Names are abbreviated, e.g., *GIR* for *GetInterestRate*. It is not customary to create parse trees for declarations, but in this case, it will facilitate semantic processing in Chapter 6.

2.6   Summary

This chapter has been a discussion of language design issues together with an example of language design. Language design is an individualistic topic. Languages are designed to meet varying criteria. Ada, for example, was designed to meet the needs of embedded system applications for the military. SmallTalk™, on which the language PSOOL concepts are modeled, was designed to facilitate top-down design of programs using abstract data types and the more recent concepts of reusability.

A new language is created by describing its syntax and semantics and becomes operational when a compiler is written to implement it. The factors which produce a popular language are: its marketing, the efficiency of its compiler, the ease with which it can be used, and other considerations.

Languages are often based upon other languages. Modula-3, for example is an object-oriented extension of Modula-2. Ada and C are somewhat Pascal-like.

2.7   Related Reading

Bergin, J. and S. Greenfield. 1988. What Does Modula-2 Need to Fully Support Object Oriented Programming?, *SIGPLAN Notices*, 23(3):73–82.
Encapsulation of data, inheritance, overloading, and message passing are shown to exist or to be easily added to the Modula-2 language.

Briot, J. and P. Cointe. 1987. A Uniform Model for Object-Oriented Languages Using the Class Abstraction, *Architectures and Languages*, 40–43.

BYTE Magazine. 1981. Special Issue on Smalltalk, *BYTE*, 6(8).

Cox, B. J. 1986. *Object Oriented Programming, An Evolutionary Approach*, Reading, MA: Addison-Wesley.
A readable and informative introductory text to object-oriented concepts.

de Champlain, M. 1990. Synapse: A Small and Expressive Object-based Real-time Programming Language, *SIGPLAN Notices*, 25(5):124–134.
Objects become tasks with concurrency implemented by asynchronous interrupt-based message passing to handlers (methods).

Demers, A., T. Reps, and T. Teitelbaum. *Attribute Propagation by Message Passing*, ACM SIGPLAN 85 Symposium on Language Issues in Programming Environments.

Donahue, J. 1990. *Modula-3: A Case Study in Programming Language Design*, SIGPLAN '90, Advanced Topics Tutorial Notes, White Plains, NY.
Discusses problems in language design, using Modula-3 as an example.

Eriksson, M. 1990. A Correct Example of Multiple Inheritance, *SIGPLAN Notices*, 25(7):7–10.

Ghezzi, C. and M. Jazayeri. 1987. *Programming Language Concepts, 2nd ed.*, New York: John Wiley & Sons.

Goldberg, A. and D. Robson. 1983. *Smalltalk-80: The Language and its Implementation.* Reading, MA: Addison-Wesley.

Harland, D. M. 1984. *Polymorphic Programming Languages, Design & Implementation*, London: Harland/Ellis Horwood Limited.

Lemone, K. A., J. J. McConnell, M. A. O'Connor, and J. Wisnewski. 1991. Implementing Semantics of Object Oriented Languages Using Attribute Grammars, *Proceedings of the ACM 19th Computer Science Conference*, San Antonio, TX.

Meyer, B. 1988. *Object-Oriented Software Construction*, Englewood Cliffs, NJ: Prentice-Hall.

Morrison, R., A. Dearle, R. C. H. Connor, and A. L. Brown. 1991. An Ad Hoc Approach to the Implementation of Polymorphism, *ACM Transactions on Programming Languages and Systems*, 13(3):342–371.

Nelson, M. L. 1991. An Objected-Oriented Tower of Babel, *OOPS Messenger*, 2(3):3–11.

Pagan, F. G. 1981. *Formal Specification of Programming Languages: A Panoramic Primer*, Englewood Cliffs, NJ: Prentice-Hall.

Schriver, B. and P. Wegner. 1988. *Research Directions in Object Oriented Programming*, Cambridge, MA: MIT Press.

Snyder, A. 1987. Encapsulation and Inheritance in Object-Oriented Programming Languages, Proc. of ACM Conf. on Object-Oriented Programming Systems, Languages and Applications, *SIGPLAN Notices,* 21(11).

U.S. Department of Defense (DOD). 1977. Requirements for High Order Computer Programming Languages, Ironman, *SIGPLAN Notices,*12(12):39–54.

U.S. Department of Defense (DOD). 1978. Requirements for High Order Computer Programming Languages, Steelman, Washington, D.C.

U.S. Department of Defense (DOD). 1980. Requirements for High Order Computer Programming Languages, Stoneman, Washington, D.C.

U.S. Department of Defense (DOD). 1983. Reference Manual for the Ada Programming Language, ANSI/MIL-STD-1815A, Washington, D.C.

Wasserman, A. I., P. A. Pircher, and R. J. Muller. 1990. The Object-Oriented Structure Design Notation for Software Design and Representation, *IEEE Computer,* 23(3):50–62.
Presents a notation for designing object-oriented systems including elements for classes and inheritance.

Wegner, P. 1987. *Dimensions of Object-Based Language Design*, OOPSLA '87, 168–182.
An excellent article for standardizing and categorizing object-based concepts.

Wilson, R. 1987. Object-Oriented Languages Reorient Programming Techniques, *Computer Design*, 52–62.

Wirth, N. 1976. *Algorithms + Data Structures = Programs*, Englewood Cliffs, NJ: Prentice-Hall

Zhai, C. 1990. Preliminary Ideas of a Conceptual Programming Language, *SIGPLAN Notices*, 25(12):93–100.

EXERCISES

1. Describe the five phases of the software system life cycle as they apply to a programming language compiler.

2. List the object-oriented concepts in PSOOL and show how they are implemented syntactically.

3. Compare PSOOL with other object-oriented languages such as C++.

4. Discuss PSOOL with respect to (a) simplicity, (b) expressiveness, and (c) orthogonality.

5. Another property of programming languages is definiteness, which is the language's ability to be precise, that is, it should be clear what is or is not a correct program. Discuss the definiteness of PSOOL.

6. PSOOL's tokens: Add Real, Character, Boolean and String literals to PSOOL production 27. Describe all of these (including integers) using a regular expression, e.g., *Integer = Digit Digit**.

7. Design regular expressions for strings and comments. (They are used in the programs!)

8. Consider how to add procedure and function calls to the PSOOL grammar. (Hint: procedure calls will be in a different production from function calls.)

PSOOL Compiler Project Part 0

The project for this text consists of writing a compiler for PSOOL. The first phase, lexical analysis, is described in the next chapter. At this point, it will be helpful to familiarize yourself with the PSOOL concepts and the BNF.

Now is also the time to decide whether you will use a tool such as LEX and YACC or whether you will write the phases yourself in a high-level language. If so, decide what language you will use.

There is a simpler project, Project II, SubAda, described in Appendix B. It describes the phases of a compiler for a small subset of Ada.

3

Scanner Generators

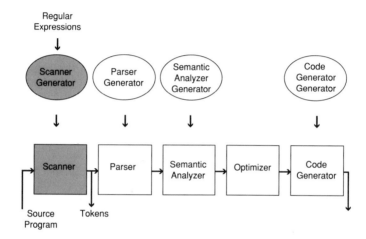

3.0 Introduction

A scanner generator, also called a lexical analyzer generator, follows the form shown in Figure 2 of Chapter 1:

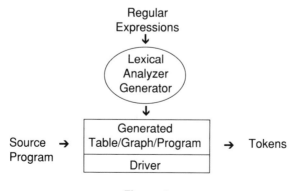

Figure 1

In Figure 1, the scanner is shown in two parts—the table or program which is generated and the driver which is written, not generated.

3.1 Metalanguage

The metalanguage for a scanner generator is a set of regular expressions describing the tokens in the language. A program stub or finite state table is generated. At compile-time, the driver reads input characters from the source program, consults the table based upon the input and the current state, and moves to a new state based upon the entry, perhaps performing an action such as entering an identifier into a name table.

We will illustrate these concepts with a sample language consisting of assignment statements whose right-hand sides are arithmetic expressions.

EXAMPLE 1   Regular expressions for the tokens in assignment statements

```
Identifier = Letter (Letter | Digit)*
Letter = A | B | ... | Z | a | b | ... | z
Digit = 0 | 1 | ... | 9
Operator = + | * | / | - | :=
Literal = Digit+
Punctuation = ; | ( | )
```

From the entries in the regular expressions in Example 1, we see that identifiers here consist of a sequence of one or more letters and digits beginning with a letter and that a literal consists of a sequence of digits. The allowable operators are those for addition, subtraction, multiplication, division and assignment.

The expression for literal uses an extended regular expression, $Digit^+$. The superscript "+" is translated as "one or more". Thus,

```
Digit+ = Digit Digit*
```

These regular expressions are input to the generator to produce state tables either in table form or as a case statement program stub.

EXAMPLE 2   Input to generator

```
Identifier    =    Letter (Letter | Digit)*
Letter        =    A | B | ... | z | a | b | ... | z
Digit         =    0 | 1 | 2 | . . . | 9
Operator      =    + | * | - | / | :=
Literal       =    Digit+
Punctuation   =    ; | ( | )
```

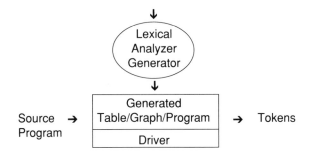

In the next sections, we discuss the two programs, the driver program and the lexical analyzer generator, itself. For the next section, we presume that the table has been created by magic, and in the following section, we will see the tedious, not so magic, algorithm for generating the table.

3.2   The Driver

For lexical analysis, we can consider the input source program as a long sequence of characters with two pointers: a *current* pointer and a *lookahead* pointer.

```
        X1 := A + Bb * 12 ;
```
Current
Lookahead

When lexical analysis begins to find the next token, *current and lookahead* both point to the same character:

```
       X1 := A + Bb * 12 ;
```
Current
Lookahead

In the algorithm, four actions will be performed on these pointers:

    (1) *GetChar*: Moves the *lookahead* pointer ahead one character and returns that character.

```
        X1 := A + Bb * 12 ;
```
Current
Lookahead

    (2) *Retract*: Moves the *lookahead* pointer back one character.

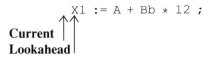

Before *Retract*   X1 := A + Bb * 12 ;

Current
Lookahead

After *Retract*   X1 := A + Bb * 12 ;

Current ──────────┘   │
Lookahead ─────────────────┘

(3) *Accept*: Moves the *current* pointer ahead to the *lookahead* pointer.

X1 := A + Bb * 12 ;

Current ↑
Lookahead

(4) *Return*: Returns a token consisting of a class and a value, as well as performs any actions associated with that state, e.g., installing an identifier
into the name table.

The driver program scans the input program and consults the entry at Table
[State,InputChar] for the new state. The entry at Table[State,InputChar] consists of a
new state and perhaps an action to be performed before moving to the new state:

Algorithm
Driver for Lexical Analysis

```
WHILE there is more input
  InputChar := GetChar
  State := Table[0, InputChar]
  WHILE State ≠ Blank
    InputChar := GetChar
    State := Table[State, InputChar]
  ENDWHILE
  Retract
  Accept
  Return token = (Class, Value )
ENDWHILE
```

In the algorithm for the lexical analysis driver, *retract* is necessary when a token
is found because the algorithm will have scanned one character too far.

Example 3 shows a piece of a state table and the execution of the algorithm on an
input string. Rows represent states, columns are input characters, and the entries in
the table are states.

EXAMPLE 3   The driver algorithm in action

State/Input	Letter	Digit	Others
0	1	2	. . .
1	1	1	all blank
. . .	. . .		

When the driver algorithm begins, the *current* and *lookahead* pointers are initialized to the character preceding the input (see Exercise 2):

```
        X1 := A + Bb * 12 ;
         ↑
Current |
Lookahead
```

The first input character, the *X*, is input (read by *GetChar*), and the next state is at Table[0,*Letter*] (see Exercise 3). The entry there is state 1. The input looks like:

```
        X1 := A + Bb * 12 ;
          ↑↑
Current | |
Lookahead
```

Since state is not blank, the algorithm enters the inner WHILE loop, and *GetChar* returns a new *InputChar,* the "1":

```
        X1 := A + Bb * 12 ;
         ↑ ↑
Current |  |
Lookahead |
```

We continue and compute a new state, the entry at Table [1, *Digit*], also equal to state 1. Thus, on encountering a digit, the lexical analyzer stays in state 1. Returning to the condition in the inner WHILE, the algorithm computes that the state is still not blank; thus *GetChar* returns the next character, either a space or, if all spaces have been removed (see Exercise 2), the ":".

```
        X1 := A + Bb * 12 ;
         ↑    ↑
Current |     |
Lookahead     |
```

There is no entry at Table[1, space] or Table[1, :], so the condition in the inner WHILE fails and the algorithm executes the statements outside the inner WHILE, first performing a *retract* operation:

```
        X1 := A + Bb * 12 ;
         ↑ ↑
Current |  |
Lookahead |
```

Then, the *accept* operation is performed, moving the *current* pointer ahead to the *lookahead* pointer:

```
        X1 := A + Bb * 12 ;
          ↑
Current
Lookahead |
```

The token *returned* is that associated with state 1, probably a token with class equal to *Id*, and a value equal to the characters in the identifier or an index into a name table where the identifier is installed (see Exercise 3).

> The lexical analyzer driver now continues with the outer WHILE loop
> until input is exhausted.

The next section discusses the lexical analyzer generator.

3.3   The Generator

Section 3.2 asks the reader to assume that the table is built by magic. The truth is that translating regular expressions to a state table or case statement is more tedious than magic. In this section, we will outline the steps and leave the algorithm to the reader (see Exercises 7 to 9).

Lexical Analyzer Generator Step 0: *Recognizing a Regular Expression*

A regular expression is either

(a) empty, representing no strings at all, denoted by ϵ, or

(b) a single letter representing the language consisting of an *A*, denoted by A, or

(c) the union of two regular expressions, such as that consisting of *A* (denoted by A) and that consisting of *B* and denoted by A | B, or

(d) the concatenation of two regular expressions, say ":" and "=", denoted ":" • "=" or, more frequently, omitting the •, as ":=", or

(e) the Kleene closure, which is the union of ϵ, with A, with A•A, with A•A•A, etc., and denoted A*.

$$A^* = \{\epsilon\} \cup A \cup A•A \cup A•A•A \cup ...$$

To convert a regular expression to a finite automaton requires the recognition of ϵ, *, | , and •, as well as the individual characters. Recognition of ϵ is not really possible, so we realize the resulting automaton will need to be converted to one which has no ϵ-transitions.

3.3.1   Lexical Analyzer Generator Step 1: *Converting a Regular Expression to a Finite Automaton*

There are five steps (a)–(e):

ϵ:

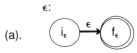

(a).

This first diagram shows that the regular expression ϵ can be recognized by the nondeterministic finite automaton which goes from its initial to its final state by reading no input. Such a move is called an ϵ-*transition*.

In table form, this would be denoted:

State/Input	ϵ ...
. . .	. . .
i	f

The reader may be wondering about an input of ϵ and how it would be recognized by the driver. In fact, it will not be. This is just a first step in table creation, and we will allow the creation of a nondeterministic finite automaton (NFA). Section 3.3.2 outlines how to turn this NFA into a deterministic finite automaton (DFA).

a:

(b).

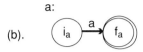

Diagram (b) shows that the language $\{a\}$ denoted by the regular expression a is recognized by the finite automaton that goes from its initial to final state by reading an a. In table form this would be:

State/Input	a
. . .	. . .
i	f

(c). $R_1 | R_2$

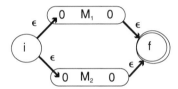

In (c), we presume that the languages denoted by the regular expressions R_1 and R_2, L_{R1} and L_{R2}, respectively, are recognized by the finite automata denoted by M_1 and M_2.

Adding ϵ-transitions to the beginning and end creates a finite automaton which will recognize either the language represented by R_1 or the language represented by R_2, i.e., the union of these two languages, $L_{R1} \cup L_{R2}$.

We could eliminate the new final state and the ϵ-transitions to it by letting the final states of M_1 and M_2 remain final states.

In table form, this is:

State/Input	$L_{R1} \cup L_{R2}$
i	. . .
. . .	f

Here, the table entry for f is shown in a different row because the process of recognizing strings in either L_{R1} or L_{R2} may lead to other intermediate states.

Our example, which recognizes

```
        Letters = A|B|C|...|a|b|...|z
and
        Literal = 0|1|2| ...|9
```

will use this step.

(d). R₁ • R₂

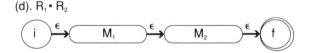

In diagram (d), M_1 is the machine that accepts L_{R1} and M_2 is the language that accepts L_{R2}. Thus, after this combined automaton has recognized a legal string in L_{R1}, it will start looking for legal strings in L_{R2}. This is exactly the set of strings denoted by $R_1 \cdot R_2$. The related table is:

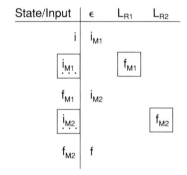

State/Input	ϵ	L_{R1}	L_{R2}
i	i_{M1}		
i_{M1}		f_{M1}	
f_{M1}	i_{M2}		
i_{M2}			f_{M2}
f_{M2}	f		

Here, the table leads from an initial state, i, to the final state of M_1 upon recognition of strings in L_{R1}, then from the final state in M_1, f_{M1} to the initial state in M_2 on an ϵ-transition, that is, without reading any input, and then from the initial state in M_2, i_{M2} to the final state in M_2, f_{M2} upon recognizing the strings in L_{R2}.

The • is often omitted. It is understood that two regular expressions appearing next to one another represents the concatenation.

We will use this step for the example, when we define an identifier as a string of letters and digits concatenated. Another example will recognize a literal as the concatenation of one or more digits, that is,

```
        Identifier = Letter (Letter | Digit)*
means
        Identifier = Letter • (Letter | Digit)*
```

(e). R*

Here, M is a finite automaton recognizing some L_R. A new initial state is added leading to both M and to a new final state. The ϵ-transition recognizes the empty string, ϵ (if R did not contain ϵ already). The transition to M causes the language L_R to be recognized. The ϵ-transition from all final states of R to its initial state will allow the recognition of L^i_R, i = 2, ... The table is:

State/Input	ϵ	L_{R1}
i	i_M,f	
i_M		f_M
f_M		
f	i	

We will use this step, as well as the preceding two, for the regular expressions

```
Identifier = Letter (Letter | Digit)*
```
and
```
Literal = Digit+ = Digit Digit*
```

Using these diagrams as guidelines, we can "build" a nondeterministic finite automaton from any regular expression (see Exercise 6).

3.3.2   Lexical Analyzer Generator Step 2: *Converting from an NFA to a DFA*

As we saw in (a) of Section 3.3.1, an NFA may have transitions on reading no input. In addition, an NFA may have more than one transition for the same input:

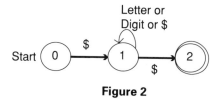

Figure 2

In Figure 2, one can go from state 1 to either state 1 or state 2 upon reading a "$".

These two possibilities, ϵ-transitions and multiple transitions on the same input, represent nondeterminism.

To convert from an NFA to a DFA, we eliminate these two possibilities by *grouping* states in the NFA. A state in the DFA will consist of a *group* (set) of states from the NFA.

The new start state is the same as the old start state.

With the new start state we group all the states we can get to upon reading the same input in the NFA; this process is continued with all the states of the NFA that are in any set of states in the DFA.

Any state in the DFA that contains a final state of the NFA is a final state.

For the NFA above, the new start state is 0', the prime to distinguish it from the old start state. State 1' = {1} since the only state accessible from state 0 in the NFA is state 1:

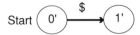

The situation is different for transitions from 1' = {1}. Upon reading a letter or a digit, the transition is back to state 1. We can add that transition to the DFA:

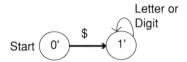

But there are two transitions upon reading "$" in the NFA, a move to state 1 and a move to state 2. We group these states into a new state called 2' = {1, 2} in the DFA. The DFA now is:

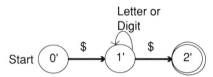

The state 2' = {1, 2} contains the old final state 2, so it is a final state.

If we are in state 2' = {1, 2} and the input is a letter or a digit, there is a transition back to 1' (because there is a transition from 1 to 1 in the NFA). Finally, there is a transition from 2' to 2' in the DFA upon reading a $ (because there is a transition from 1 to 1 upon reading a $ in the NFA and 2' = {1, 2}). The final DFA is:

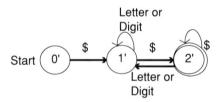

This step of the lexical analyzer generator, conversion of a regular expression to a DFA, has shown the automata in state-transition form. This could equally well have been shown in table form (see Exercise 7).

The step for removing ε-transitions is similar; all the states accessible via an ε-transition are grouped (see Exercise 6). This step can frequently result in DFA's with many states, some of which are performing the same function and can be combined. This is a necessary step in generating a lexical analyzer since there may be hundreds of states in the table for the tokens in a programming language.

A purist would not consider the above automaton a true DFA since a true DFA will have a transition somewhere upon reading any character in the alphabet. Thus, state 0' should have an arrow (leading to an "error" state) upon reading a letter or a digit.

3.3.3   Lexical Analyzer Generator Step 3: *Conversion to a Minimal DFA*

Minimizing a DFA consists of merging states which perform the same action. They can be found by repeated *partitioning*. We will show this for an NFA in table form. Final states 2 and 4 are shown in boldface:

State/Input	Letter or Digit	$
start 0	−	1
1	3	2
2	5	4
3	5	4
4	3	4
5	3	4

The first step is to partition the table into final and non-final states:

State/Input	Letter or Digit	$
start 0	−	1
1	3	2
3	5	4
5	3	4
2	5	4
4	3	4

The partitioning continues by partitioning out states that lead to the same partition for the same input. Here, states 1, 3, and 5 lead to the last partitioned state upon reading a "$", while state 0 does not, so we put state 0 into a new partition:

State/Input	Letter or Digit	$
start 0	−	1
1	3	2
3	5	4
5	3	4
2	5	4
4	3	4

All states in the second partition go to the same partition upon reading a letter or digit, and they all go to the third partition upon reading a "$". Thus, we are done, and relabeling the state table yields:

State/Input	Letter or Digit	$
start 0	−	1
1	1	2
2	1	2

This concludes the minimization step (see Exercise 8) and the procedure for conversion of a regular expression to a minimal finite automaton, that is, we have described a lexical analyzer generator.

3.4   Error Handling

The only errors appropriately handled by a lexical analyzer are those which misuse a sequence of characters. Errors such as using a reserved word as an identifier are syntax errors to be found by the parser.

One way to handle errors is to define error tokens. For example, if the language does not contain a ".", a regular expression can be defined using one and the associated action would be to report an error.

Anticipating user errors has met with limited success.

3.5   Generating a Lexical Analyzer vs. Writing a Lexical Analyzer

The reader may think it is much harder to write a lexical analyzer generator than it is just to write a lexical analyzer and then make changes to it to produce a different lexical analyzer. After all, most programming languages have similar tokens. This thought has been voiced by many compiler experts. In fact, many compiler tools allow the user to write a lexical analyzer and call it from the generated parser or to make changes to a lexical analyzer provided by the tool.

Nevertheless, the process is informative, and there may be applications for which the user may wish to be able to generate various lexical analyzers.

The next section shows an example of a lexical analyzer generator, LEX (Lesk and Schmidt, 1975), a tool which comes with UNIX.

3.6   LEX, A Lexical Analyzer Generator

This section describes LEX, a lexical analyzer generator, written by Lesk and Schmidt at Bell Labs in 1975 for the UNIX operating system. It now exists for many operating systems, and versions can be obtained for almost any system including microcomputers. The discussion here is for illustration and should not be considered sufficient to use LEX.

LEX produces a scanner which is a C program (there is also a RatFOR version) that can be compiled and linked with other compiler modules. Other LEX-like tools exist which generate lexical analyzers in Pascal, Ada, etc.

LEX accepts regular expressions and allows actions, code to be executed, to be associated with each regular expression. At scan time, when an input string matches one of the defined regular expressions, the action code is executed.

3.6.1   The LEX Metalanguage

The LEX metalanguage input consists of three parts: (1) definitions which give names to sequences of characters, (2) translation rules which define tokens and allow association of a number representing the class, and (3) user-written procedures in C which are associated with a regular expression. Each of the three sections is separated by a double percent sign, "%%". The input has the following form:

```
Definitions  ← Gives names to sequences of characters
%%
Rules  ← Defines tokens. Class may be returned as a #
%%
User-Written Procedures  ←  In C
```

The definitions section consists of a sequence of *Names,* each followed by an expression to be given that name.

The rules consist of a sequence of regular expressions, each followed by an (optional) action which returns a number for that regular expression and performs other actions if desired, such as installing the characters in the token in a table.

The user-written procedures are the code for the C functions invoked as actions in the rules. Thus, the form for each section is:

```
Name1           Expression1
Name2           Expression2
...
%%
RegExp1         {Action1}
RegExp2         {Action2}
...
%%
C function1
C function2
...
```

A section may be empty, but the "%%" is still needed.

Like UNIX itself, the metalanguage is case-sensitive, that is, "A" and "a" are read as different characters.

Example 4 shows a LEX description for our language consisting of assignment statements. There are other ways of expressing the tokens described here.

EXAMPLE 4   Assignment statement language tokens in LEX

```
/* Definitions */

Delimiter       [ \t\n]
WhiteSpace      {Delimiter}+
Letter          [A-Za-z]
Digit           [0-9]

%%

/* Translation rules */

{Letter}({Letter} | {Digit})*
        {printf ("\t(Id,",%S")\n",yytext);return(Id)}

{Digit}+
     {printf ("\t(Lit,",%S")\n",yytext);return(Lit)}

("+"|"-"|"*"|"/"|":=")
        {printf ("\t(Op,",%S")\n",yytext);return(Op)}

(";" | "(" | ")" )
{printf ("\t(Punct,",%S")\n",yytext);return(Punct)}

%%
```

In Example 4, a delimiter is defined to be a space or a tab or a new-line character. Tab is denoted "\t", and carriage return is "\n". WhiteS-pace is one or more delimiter. No user-written procedures are shown. There are other ways to find these same tokens using LEX.

3.6.2 Functionality of LEX

The C code scanner generated by LEX can be altered before it is compiled. The generated scanner is actually written to be "parser-driven"; when it is integrated into a compiler front end, it is invoked by the parser.

Figure 3 shows how the tool operates. These steps may vary from system to system:

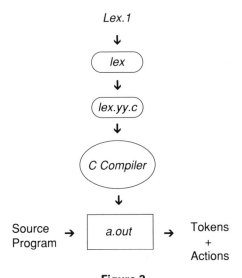

Figure 3

The LEX metalanguage description is input in a file called *lex.1*. LEX produces a file called *lex.yy.c*. The generated lexical analyzer is in UNIX's executable file called *a.out*.

Within the generated *lex.yy.c* is a C function called *yylex()* which performs *GetChar* and the other actions discussed in Section 3.2.

The resulting scanner matches the longest input sequence. If a keyword is defined, say "If", and an identifier "IfName" is used, the identifier "IfName" will be found.

If two regular expressions match a particular input, then the first one defined is used.

There are many more details of LEX's functionality to be described, and the reader is invited to look at a user's manual for any available LEX to which he or she may have access.

3.7 Summary

This has been an introduction to lexical analyzer generators and the process of converting from a regular expression to a minimal DFA. This conversion is so complicated that many computer scientists advocate writing a lexical analyzer and then making changes to it for new applications. This works well for applications where the tokens are quite similar.

The process of generating a lexical analyzer has been likened to the compiler process itself:

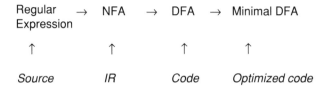

There are several lexical analyzer generators on the market, making it unlikely that anyone except a compiler tool designer or a student in a sadistic instructor's class would ever have to write one.

3.8 Related Reading

Bickel, M. A. 1987. Automatic Correction to Misspelled Names: A Fourth Generation Language Approach, *CACM*, 30:224–228.

Chapman, N. 1989. Regular Attribute Grammars and Finite State Machines, *SIGPLAN Notices*, 24(6):97–104.

Johnson, W. L., J. H. Porter, S. I. Ackley, and D. T. Ross. 1968. Automatic Generation of Efficient Lexical Processors using Finite-State Machines, *CACM*, 11(12):805–813.

Background Reading

Holub, A. 1990. *Compiler Design in C*, Englewood Cliffs, NJ: Prentice-Hall.

Hopcroft, J. E. and J. D. Ullman. 1979. *Introduction to Automata Theory, Languages and Computation*, Reading, MA: Addison-Wesley.

Lesk, M. E. and E. Schmidt. 1975. *LEX: A Lexical Analyzer Generator*, in UNIX Programmer's Manual 2, Murray Hill, NJ: AT&T Bell Laboratories.

EXERCISES

1. Write regular expressions for:
   (a) Real numbers that include those represented by the following examples: 0.3, 3.0, 1.52, 0.5E-1.
   (b) Identifiers that begin and end with $ and have any number of letters, digits, and $ in between.
   (c) Relational operators as expressed in:
      (i)   Pascal: <, >, =, <>, <=, >=
      (ii) FORTRAN: .LT., .GT., .EQ., .NE., .LE., .GE.
      (iii) Ada: =, /=, <, <=, >, >=
      (iv) A language of your choice

2. The driver algorithm in Section 3.2 is missing many details. For example, the issue of blanks needs to be addressed. Extend the algorithm to ignore blanks and to:

   (a) Use blanks as a delimiter within the strings, that is, finding a blank denotes the end of the current token.

   (b) Allow blanks within tokens, that is, *Max 1* is the same token as *Max1*.

3. Example 3 shows a partial table for recognizing an identifier consisting of letters and digits beginning with a letter. Since neither letter nor digit is a single character, more details need to be provided. Traditionally there have been two methods. Discuss what these might be (and then check the answers to selected exercises).

4. Show a CASE statement equivalent to the table in Example 3.

5. Write the details of the four actions *GetChar, Accept, Retract, and Return* from Section 3.2.

6. From the method described in Section 3.3.1, write an algorithm to convert from a regular expression to an NFA. Describe the NFA as an abstract data type, rather than deciding upon a particular implementation such as a table or CASE statement.

7. Using the method described in step 2 of Section 3.3.2, write an algorithm to convert from an NFA to a DFA, again describing each of the NFA's as an abstract data type.

8. Using the method described in step 2 of Section 3.3.3, write an algorithm to convert from a DFA to a minimal DFA, again describing each of the DFA's as an abstract data type.

9. Implement an NFA (as described in Exercises 6 and 7) as (a) a table and (b) a CASE statement.

10. Name some applications where it would be better to do the extensive work required to write a lexical analyzer generator, rather than writing a lexical analyzer and then making changes to it when needed.

11. Is the LEX grammar unstratified? You will need a LEX manual to answer this.

12. The table in Section 3.3.1 step (d) is incomplete. Add the missing information.

PSOOL Compiler Project Part 1

Lexical Analysis

Time: 20–30 hours

Using the grammar for PSOOL actions, select one of the following three options.

The grammar is found in Figure 1 of Chapter 2, Section 2.2. Since we are not implementing the class declarations in this assignment, you may wish to change the first production to:

```
Program → {Action}⁺
```

Option 1 (Easier):   Using a compiler tool such as LEX, code the regular expressions for the tokens and generate a lexical analyzer.

Option 2 (Easier):   Make the necessary changes to a given lexical analyzer (many tools include one) to find the tokens.

Option 3 (Much, much harder):   Using the methods of this chapter and the algorithms from Exercises 2 to 9, write a lexical analyzer generator.

Run your lexical analyzer on the following input:

```
(a)  Action One;
    LocalNames a, b,c,xyz,p,q : Integer;
    BeginAction
        a := b3;
        xyz := a + b + c
             - p / q;
        a := xyz * (p + q);
        p := a - xyz - p;
    endaction;

(b)  Action Two;
    LocalNames i,j : Integer;
    BeginAction
        If i > j Then
            i := i + j;
        Elsif i < j Then
            i := 1;
        End if;
    EndAction;

(c)  Action Three;
    LocalNames i,j,k : Integer;
    BeginAction
        while (i < j) And (j < k) Loop
            k := k + 1;
            While (i = j) Loop
                i := i + 2;
            End Loop;
        End Loop;
    EndAction;

(d)  Action CreateNewSavingsAccount;
    LocalNames
        CompoundInterestRate := 6;
        ThisAccount: SavingsAccount;
        IO : Utilities;
    BeginAction
        ThisAccount :=  New (SavingsAccount);
        IO :=  New (Utilities);
        IO : PutPrompt ("Owner?");
        IO : Input (Owner);
```

```
    ThisAccount : SetOwner(Owner);
    IO : PutPrompt ("Address?");
    IO : Input (Address);
    ThisAccount : SetAddress (Address);
    IO : PutPrompt ("PhoneNumber?");
    IO : Input (PhoneNumber);
    ThisAccount:
       SetPhoneNumber(PhoneNumber);
    ThisAccount : GenerateAccountNumber;
    IO : PutPrompt ("InitialDeposit");
    IO : Input (InitialDeposit);
    ThisAccount : DepositFunds
         (InitialDeposit);
    ThisAccount : AddInterestToBalance;
EndAction CreateNewSavingsAccount;
```

```
(e)  Action AddInterest;
LocalNames
Account1 : NOWAccount;
Account2 : SavingsAccount;
IO : Utilities;
BeginAction
   IO := New(Utilities);
   IO : Input(AccountName);
   Account1 :=
   Get(NOWAccount);
Account2 :=
   Get(SavingsAccount);
   Account1 : AddInterestToBalance;
   Account2 : AddInterestToBalance;
EndAction AddInterest;
```

```
(e)  Action AddInterest;
LocalNames
Account: BankAccount;
IO : Utilities;
BeginAction
IO := New(Utilities);
IO : Input(AccountType);
IO : Input(AccountName);
IO: Input(Deposit);
Account := New(AccountType);
Account : DepositFunds(Deposit);
Account : AddInterestToBalance;
EndAction AddInterest;
```

```
(f) A program of your choice.
```

4

Top-Down Parser Generators

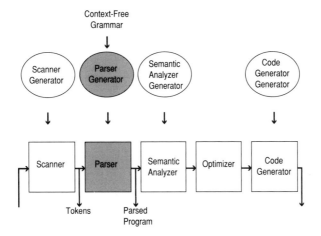

4.0   Introduction

A parser generator, also called a syntax analyzer generator, follows the form shown in Chapter 1, Figure 3:

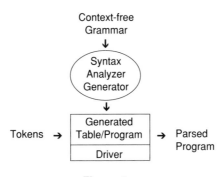

Figure 1

Although syntax analysis is more powerful than lexical analysis (a parser can recognize tokens), it is not necessarily more complicated to generate one. In fact, generation of a top-down parser is relatively simple.

4.1   Metalanguage for Top-Down Parser Generation

The metalanguage for a parser generator is a context-free grammar. This context-free grammar is usually expressed in Backus-Naur form, BNF, or extended Backus-Naur form, EBNF (see PSOOL Project Part 2 at the end of the chapter), themselves metalanguages for context-free grammars. EBNF differs from BNF, allowing shortcuts resulting in fewer but more complicated productions. In this text, we often say the metalanguage for a parser generator is BNF.

EXAMPLE 1   BNF for assignment statement program

```
Program       → Statements
Statements    → Statement Statements
                | Statement
Statement     → AsstStmt ;
AsstStmt      → Id := Expression
Expression    → Term Expression'
Expression'   → + Term Expression'
                | ε
Term          →  Factor Term'
Term'         → * Factor Term'
                | ε
Factor        → (Expression)
                | Id
                | Lit
```

The BNF shown in Example 1 states that a program consists of a sequence of statements, each of which is an assignment statement with a right-hand side consisting of an arithmetic expression. This BNF is input to the parser generator to produce tables which are then accessed by the driver as the input is read.

This BNF is more complicated than that shown in Chapter 1 for parser generation. Top-down parser generation places more restrictions on the grammar. In the next sections, we convert the grammar of Chapter 1 to this form.

EXAMPLE 2   Input to parser generator

```
Program       → Statements
Statements    → Statement
                | Statement Statements
Statement     → AsstStmt ;
AsstStmt      → Id := Expression
Expression    → Term Expression'
Expression'   → + Term Expression'
                | ε
```

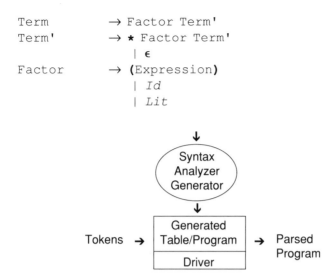

```
Term        → Factor Term'
Term'       → * Factor Term'
            | ε
Factor      → (Expression)
            | Id
            | Lit
```

The parser generator converts the BNF into tables. The form of the tables depends upon whether the generated parser is a top-down parser or a bottom-up parser. Top-down parsers are easy to generate; bottom-up parsers are more difficult to generate.

4.1.1 Metalanguage Restrictions

The grammar from Chapters 1 and 2 actually has two problems which the parser generator must eliminate. We discuss these as preprocessor steps to the parser generator.

Left-Recursion

The grammar for assignment statements from Chapters 1 and 2 is left-recursive; in the process of expanding the first nonterminal, that nonterminal is generated again:

$$\text{Expression} \rightarrow \text{Expression} + \text{Term}$$
$$\uparrow \qquad\qquad \uparrow$$

The most reasonable top-down parsing method is one where we look only at the next token in the input. Looking at more than the next token has proved too time-consuming in practice. Parsing, here initiated by the driver program, proceeds by expanding productions until a terminal (token) is finally generated. Then that terminal is read from the input and the procedure continues. If the first nonterminal is the same as that being expanded, as in the production for an expression above, it will be continually and infinitely expanded without ever generating a terminal that can be matched in the grammar.

Generation of top-down parsers may require a preprocessing step that eliminates left-recursion.

Common Prefix

A second problem is caused by two productions for the same nonterminal whose right-hand side begins with the same symbol:

$$S \rightarrow a \ \alpha$$
$$\rightarrow a \ \beta$$

These two productions contain a *common prefix*, and once again the parser, as initiated by the driver looking at only the next symbol in the input, does not know which of these productions to choose. Fortunately, grammars can be changed to eliminate these problems. We will show algorithms for changing the grammars to eliminate both left-recursion and common prefixes.

4.1.2   Elimination of Left-Recursion

There is a formal technique for eliminating left-recursion from productions:

Step One: Direct-Recursion

For each rule which contains a left-recursive option,

$$A \rightarrow A \ \alpha \ | \ \beta$$

introduce a new nonterminal A' and rewrite the rule as

$$A \rightarrow \beta \ A'$$
$$A' \rightarrow \epsilon \ | \ \alpha \ A'$$

Thus the production:

$$E \rightarrow E + T \ | \ T$$

is left-recursive with "E" playing the role of A, "+ T" playing the role of α, and "T" playing the role of β. Introducing the new nonterminal E', the production can be replaced by:

$$E \rightarrow T \ E'$$
$$E' \rightarrow \epsilon \ | + T \ E'$$

Of course, there may be more than one left-recursive part on the right-hand side. The general rule is to replace

$$A \rightarrow A\alpha_1 \ | \ A\alpha_2 \ | \ A\alpha_3 \ | \ldots | \ A\alpha_n \ | \ \beta_1 \ | \ \beta_2 \ | \ldots | \ \beta_m$$

by

$$A \rightarrow \ \beta_1 A' \ | \ \beta_2 A' \ | \ldots | \ \beta_m A'$$
$$A' \rightarrow \epsilon \ | \ \alpha_1 A' \ | \ \alpha_2 A' \ | \ldots | \ \alpha_n A'$$

Note that this may change the "structure". For the expressions above, the original grammar is left-associative, while the non-left-recursive one is now right-associative.

Step Two: Indirect Recursion

Step one describes a rule to eliminate direct left recursion from a production. To eliminate left-recursion from an entire grammar may be more difficult because of indirect left-recursion. For example,

```
A → B x y | x
B → C  D
C → A | c
D→ d
```

is indirectly recursive because $A \to B\ x\ y \to C\ D\ x\ y \to A\ D\ x\ y$. That is, $A \to \ldots \to$ $A\ \omega$ where ω is "D x y".

The following algorithm eliminates left-recursion entirely. It contains a "call" to a procedure which eliminates direct left-recursion (as described in step one).

Algorithm
EliminateLeftRecursion

```
Arrange the nonterminals in some order, A₁, A₂,
A₃, ... Aₙ.
 FOR i := 1 TO n DO
 BEGIN {FOR i}
  FOR j := 1 TO n DO
  BEGIN {FOR j}
    (1) Replace each production of the form Aᵢ → Aⱼγ
        by the productions:
```

$$A_i \to \delta_1\gamma \mid \delta_2\gamma \mid \ldots \mid \delta_k\gamma$$

```
    where:
```

$$A_j \to \delta_1 \mid \delta_2 \mid \ldots \mid \delta_k$$

```
        are all the current Aⱼ - productions.
    (2) Eliminate the direct left recursion from the Aᵢ
        productions
  END {FOR j}
 END {FOR i}
```

We will illustrate this algorithm for the grammar above.

EXAMPLE 3   Eliminating left-recursion

Arrange the nonterminals in some order: $A_1 = A$, $A_2 = B$, $A_3 = C$, $A_4 = D$

i := 1, j := 1 :   (1) No productions of the form A → Aγ
                    (2) No direct left-recursion for A

i := 1, j := 2 :   (1) Replace A → B x y with A → C D x y
                    (2) Still no direct left-recursion for A

i := 1, j := 3 :   (1) Replace A → C D x y with A → A D x y and
                        A → c D x y

                    (2) Eliminate direct left-recursion for A → A D x y
                        Replace with A → c D x y A'
                        A → x A'
                        A' → ε | D x y A'

i := 1, j := 3 :   (1) No productions of the form A → Dγ
                   (2) No direct left-recursion for A

I := 2, j := 1 :   (1) No productions of the form B → Aγ
                   (2) No direct left-recursion for B

I := 2, j := 2 :   (1) No productions of the form B → Bγ
                   (2) No direct left-recursion for B

I := 2, j := 3 :   (1) Replace B → C D with B → A D and B → c D
                   (2) No direct left-recursion for B

I := 2, j := 4 :   (1) No productions of the form B → Dγ
                   (2) No direct left-recursion for B

I := 3, j := 1 :   (1) Replace C → A with C → c D x y A'
                       C → x A'
                   (2) No direct left-recursion for C

I := 3, j := 2 :   (1) No productions of the form C → Bγ
                   (2) No direct left-recursion for C

I := 3, j := 3 :   (1) No productions of the form C → Cγ
                   (2) No direct left-recursion for C

I := 3, j := 4 :   (1) No productions of the form C → Dγ
                   (2) No direct left-recursion for D

I := 4, j := 1 :   (1) No productions of the form D → Aγ
                   (2) No direct left-recursion for D

I := 4, j := 2 :   (1) No productions of the form D → Bγ
                   (2) No direct left-recursion for D

I := 4, j := 3 :   (1) No productions of the form D → γ
                   (2) No direct left-recursion for D

I := 4, j := 4 :   (1) No productions of the form D → Dγ
                   (2) No direct left-recursion for D

The resulting grammar is

A → c D x y A'
A → x A'
A' → ε | D x y A'
B → A D
B → c D
C → c D x y A'
C → x A'
D → d

4.1.3   Elimination of Common Prefixes

The procedure to eliminate a common prefix is called *left-factoring*.

The formal technique is quite simple. Simply change

$$A \rightarrow \beta \, \alpha_1 \mid \beta\alpha_2 \ldots \mid \beta\alpha_n$$

to

$$A \rightarrow \beta \, A'$$
$$A' \rightarrow \alpha_1 \mid \alpha_2 \ldots \mid \alpha_n$$

In the next two sections we describe the driver algorithm and the parser generator for a top-down parser. Once again, we presume that the tables are created by magic, in order to concentrate on the driver algorithm. By now, the reader knows that the magic will ultimately change to an algorithm for generating the table.

4.2   LL(1) Parser Driver

Top-down parsing proceeds by expanding productions, beginning with the start symbol. The method shown here is for generation of an *LL(1)* parser.

In order to define LL(1), we need two preliminary definitions: FIRST and FOLLOW. FIRST is defined for a sentential form; FOLLOW is defined for a nonterminal.

FIRST(α) , for any sentential form α, is the set of terminals that begin any string derivable from α including ϵ if ϵ is derivable from α.

For a nonterminal A in a sentential form, say $\omega_1 A\omega_2$, where ω_1 and ω_2 are some string of terminals and nonterminals,

FOLLOW(A) = FIRST(ω_2)

That is, FOLLOW(A) is the set of terminals that can appear to the right of A in a sentential form.

A grammar is LL(1) if and only if given any two productions $A \rightarrow \alpha$, $A \rightarrow \beta$,

(a)   FIRST(α) $\cap$ FIRST(β) = ϕ, and

(b)   If one of α or β derives ϵ, say

$$\alpha \rightarrow \ldots \rightarrow \epsilon$$

then FIRST(β) $\cap$ FOLLOW(A) = ϕ,

Elimination of left-recursion and left-factoring aid in producing an LL(1) grammar.

If the grammar is LL(1), we need only examine the next token to decide which production to use. The magic table contains a production at the entry for Table[Nonterminal,Input Token].

Top-down parsing uses a stack of symbols, initialized to the start symbol.

Algorithm
LL(1) Parser Driver

```
Push a $ on the stack.
Initialize the stack to the start symbol.
REPEAT  WHILE stack is nonempty:
  CASE top of the stack is:

  terminal: IF input symbol matches terminal, THEN
            advance input and pop stack, ELSE error

  nonterminal: Use nonterminal and current input
               symbol to find correct production
               in table.
               Pop stack.
               Push right-hand side of production
                 from table onto stack, last symbol
                 first.
END REPEAT
IF input is finished, THEN accept, ELSE error
```

EXAMPLE 4   LL(1) parsing

Using the assignment grammar from Example 2 with the following abbreviations :

```
P = Program
U = Statements
S = Statement
A = AssignmentStatement
E = Expression
T = Term
F = Factor
```

and with left-recursion and common prefixes removed:

```
P → U
U → S U'
U'→ ε | U
S → A ;
A → Id := E
E → T E'
E'→ + T E' | ε
T → F T'
T'→ * F T' | ε
F → (E) | Id
```

The (magically created) table is shown on the following page. The table contains a row for each nonterminal and a column for each terminal. Here, we show only the part of the token needed to make the decision. All *Id* tokens are the same, but operator tokens have to be shown individually, since the parse is different for different operators.

TERMINALS

NONTERMINALS		ID	+	*	(	)	;	$
	P	P → U						
	U	U → SU'						
	U'	U' → U						U' → ε
	S	S → A ;						
	E	E → TE'			E → TE'			
	E'		E' → +TE'			E' → ε	E' → ε	E' → ε
	T	T → FT'			T → FT'			
	T'		T' → ε	T' → *FT'		T' → ε	T' → ε	T' → ε
	F	F → Id			F → (E)			

The input string is:

```
a := b * c + d ;
```

Following the steps in the algorithm:

(1) P is first pushed onto the stack. Since there is now a nonterminal on the top of the stack, the choice of nonterminal in the Case statement is taken. The current input symbol is *a*, which is an *Id*. We therefore consult the table at Table[P,Id] which contains the production P → U. In (2), we replace the P at the top of the stack with U:

Stack	**Input**	**Production**
(1) $ P	a := b * c + d ; $	P → U
(2) $ U	a := b * c + d ; $	

With the top of stack, U, we consult the table at Table [U, a]. The production there is U → S U'. We pop the top of the stack and replace it with S U' (with S on the "top"):

(2) $ U	a := b * c + d ; $	U → S U'
(3) $ U' S	a := b * c + d ; $	

Continuing,

$ U' S	a := b * c + d ; $	S → A ;
$ U' ; A	a := b * c + d ; $	A → Id := E
$ U' ; E := Id	a := b * c + d ; $	

Now, the terminal option in the CASE statement is chosen since the top of the stack contains a terminal. This is matched with the first terminal in the input, and the stack is popped as the input is advanced:

$ U' ; E :=	:= b * c + d ; $

The top of the stack is a terminal which matches the input. The stack and input become:

```
$ U' ; E                    b * c + d ; $
```

Continuing,

```
$ U' ; E                    a * b + c ; $          E → T E'
$ U' ; E' T                 a * b + c ; $          T → F T'
$ U' ; E' T' F              a * b + c ; $          F → Id
$ U' ; E' T' Id             a * b + c ; $
$ U' ; E' T'                  * b + c ; $          T'→ * F T'
$ U' ; E' T' F *              * b + c ; $
$ U' ; E' T' F                 b + c ; $           F → Id
$ U' ; E' T' Id                b + c ; $
$ U' ; E' T'                     + c ; $           T'→ ε
$ U' ; E'                        + c ; $           E'→ + T E'
$ U' ; E' T +                    + c ; $
$ U' ; E' T                        c ; $           T → F T'
$ U' ; E' T' F                     c ; $           F → Id
$ U' ; E' T' Id                   Id ; $
$ U' ; E' T'                         ; $           T'→ ε
$ U' ; E'                            ; $           E'→ ε
$ U' ;                               ; $
$ U'                                   $           U'→ ε
$                                      $
Accept!
```

Since we have run out of input exactly when the stack became empty, the input string is one of the strings accepted by the grammar. If we construct a derivation using the productions in the Production column, we will construct a left-most derivation.

4.3 Generating LL(1) Parsing Tables

Constructing LL(1) parsing tables is relatively easy (compared to constructing the tables for lexical analysis). The table is constructed using the following algorithm:

Algorithm
LL(1) Table Generation
For every production A → α in the grammar:

1. If α can derive a string starting with a (i.e., for all a in FIRST(α)),

   Table[A, a] = A → α

2. If α can derive the empty string, ε, then, for all b that can follow a string derived from A (i.e., for all b in FOLLOW(A)),

   Table[A, b] = A → α

Undefined entries are set to error, and, if any entry is defined more than once, then the grammar is *not* LL(1).

EXAMPLE 5   Constructing an LL(1) parse table entry using rule 1

Consider the production E → TE' from the non-left-recursive, left-factored expression grammar in Example 4. FIRST(TE') = {(, Id}, so Table[E,( ] = E → TE' and Table[E,Id] = E → TE' (see preceding table).

EXAMPLE 6   Constructing an LL(1) parse table entry using rule 2

Consider the production E' → ε from the same grammar of Example 4. Since ";", ")" and "$" are in FOLLOW(E'), this production occurs in the table in the row labeled E', and the columns labeled ";", ")" , and "$".

LL(1) parsing tables may be generated automatically by writing procedures for FIRST(α) and FOLLOW(A). Then, when the grammar is input, A and α are identified for each production and the two steps above followed to create the table.

4.4   Recursive Descent Parsing

LL(1) parsing is often called "table-driven recursive descent". *Recursive descent parsing* uses recursive procedures to model the parse tree to be constructed. For each nonterminal in the grammar, a procedure, which parses a nonterminal, is constructed. Each of these procedures may read input, match terminal symbols or call other procedures to read input and match terminals in the right-hand side of a production.

Consider the Assignment Statement Grammar from Example 1:

```
Program       → Statements
Statements    → Statement Statements'
Statements'   → ε | Statements
Statement     → AsstStmt ;
AsstStmt      → Id := Expression
Expression    → Term Expression'
Expression'   → + Term Expression'
              | ε
Term          → Factor Term'
Term'         → * Factor Term'
              | ε
Factor        → (Expression)
              | Id
              | Lit
```

In recursive descent parsing, the grammar is thought of as a program with each production as a (recursive) procedure. Thus, there would be a procedure corresponding to the nonterminal *Program*. It would process the right-hand side of the production. Since the right-hand side of the production is itself a nonterminal, the body of the the procedure corresponding to *Program* (we have called it *P*) will consist of a call to the procedure corresponding to *Statements* (called *Ss*). Roughly, the procedures are as follows:

```
Procedure P
BEGIN {P}
 Call Ss    {Statements}
 PRINT ("P found")
END {P}
```

The procedure corresponding to *Statements* also consists of calls corresponding to the nonterminals on the right-hand side of the production:

```
Procedure Ss
BEGIN {Ss}
 Call S  {Statement}
 Call Ss' {Statements'}
 PRINT ("Ss found")
END {Ss}
```

Skipping to the procedure corresponding to *AsstStatement*:

```
Procedure A
BEGIN {A}
  IF NextToken = "Id" THEN
    BEGIN
    PRINT ("Id found")
    Advance past it
    IF NextToken =  ":=" THEN
      BEGIN {IF}
        PRINT (":= found")
        Advance past it
        Call  E
        END {IF}
    END
PRINT ("A found")
END {A}
```

Procedures E and E' would be:

```
Procedure E
BEGIN {E}
 Call T
 Call E'
 PRINT ("E found")
END {E}

Procedure E'
BEGIN {E'}
  IF NextSymbol in input = "+" THEN
  BEGIN {IF}
    PRINT ("+ found")
    Advance  past it
    Call T
    Call E'
```

```
        PRINT ("E' found")
      END {IF}
    END {E'}
```

This procedure works fine for correct programs since it presumes that if "+" is not found, then the production is E' → ε.

Procedures T and T' are similar since the grammar productions for them are similar. Procedure F could be written:

```
        Procedure F
        BEGIN {F}
        CASE NextSymbol is
"(" :   PRINT ("(found")
        Advance past it
        Call E
        IF NextSymbol = ")" THEN
        BEGIN {IF}
          PRINT (") found")
          Advance past it
          PRINT ("F found")
        END {IF}
        ELSE
          error
"Id":         PRINT ("Id found")
              Advance past it
              PRINT ("F found")
Otherwise: error
        END {F}
```

Here, *NextSymbol* is the token produced by the lexical analyzer. To advance past it, a call to get the next token might be made. The PRINT statements will print out the reverse of a left derivation and then the parse tree can be drawn by hand or a procedure can be written to stack up the information and print it out as a real left-most derivation, indenting to make the levels of the "tree" clearer.

Recursive descent parsing has the same restrictions as the general LL(1) parsing method described earlier. Recursive descent parsing is the method of choice when the language is LL(1), when there is no tool available, and when a quick compiler is needed. Turbo Pascal is a recursive descent parser.

4.5   Error Handling in LL(1) Parsing

Much work has been done in error handling for parser generators. Some perform a *recovery* process so that parsing may continue; a few try to *repair* the error. Top-down parsers *detect* the erroneous token when it is shifted onto the stack. An error *report* might be

        Unexpected *erroneous token*

with the parser driver attempting a recovery based upon the choices that would have been valid instead of the erroneous token. The attempted recovery, adding or deleting tokens, may be made to either the stack or the input.

Error handling similar to that used for recursive descent parsing may be added to the driver. Adding error handling to recursive descent parsing is described in Lemone (1992). The method was developed by Niklaus Wirth in 1976. It requires that a set of *firsts* and *followers* be maintained or computed for each production.

4.6   Summary

This chapter discusses top-down parser generators.

Given a grammar which is LL(1), it is easy to use an LL(1) parser generator. It is even easy to write an LL(1) parser generator.

If the underlying language is LL(1), but the grammar is not, that is, it contains left-recursion or common prefixes, then the grammar must be changed, a fairly complicated process.

If the language is not LL(1), however, bottom-up parsing techniques may need to be used.

4.7   Related Reading

Aho, A., S. C. Johnson, and J. D. Ullman. 1975. Deterministic Parsing of Ambiguous Grammars, *CACM*, 18(8):441–452.

Brown, P. J. 1983. Error Messages: The Neglected Area of Man/Machine Interface, *CACM*, 26(4):246–249.

Burke, M. and G. A. Fisher. 1982. A Practical Method for Syntactic Error Diagnosis and Repair, *SIGPLAN Notices*, 17(6):67–78.

Dobler, H. and K. Pirklbauer, 1990. Coco-2: A New Compiler Compiler, *SIGPLAN Notices*, 25(5):82–90.

Uses separate metalanguages for scanner generation and parser/evaluator generation, but within the same file, producing a Modula-2 scanner and top-down parser with inherited and synthesized attribute evaluation via Modula-2 parameters and procedures.

Donahue, J. 1990. *Modula-3: A Case Study in Programming Language Design*, SIGPLAN '90 Advanced Topics Tutorial.

Discusses problems in language design, using Modula-3 as an example.

Fischer, C. N., J. Mauney, and D. R. Milton. 1980. Efficient LL(1) Error Correction and Recovery Using only Insertions, *Acta Informatica*, 13(2):141–154.

Fischer, C. N. and R. J. LeBlanc, Jr. 1988. *Crafting a Compiler*, Menlo Park, CA: Benjamin/ Cummings.

Contains an entire chapter on error handling for top-down and bottom-up parsers.

Genillard, C. and A. Strohmeier. 1988. GRAMOL: A Grammar Description Language for Lexical and Syntactic Parsers, *SIGPLAN Notices*, 23(10):103–122.

Using Ada packages for implementation, and an unstratified metalanguage, scanners and either top-down or bottom-up parsers are produced, allowing for a dynamic change of source language.

Hammond, K. and V. J. Rayward-Smith. 1984. A Survey on Syntactic Error Recovery and Repair, *Computer Languages*, 9(7):51–67.

Holub, A. 1990. *Compiler Design in C*, Englewood Cliffs, NJ: Prentice-Hall.

Contains a complete description, right down to a user manual and the C code for a top-down parser generator and a bottom-up parser generator.

Knuth, D. E. 1971. Top-down Syntax Analysis, *Acta Informatica*, 1(2):79–110.

Lemone, K. A. 1992. *Fundamentals of Compilers*, Boca Raton, FL: CRC Press.

Mauney, J. and C. N. Fischer. 1988. Determining the Extent of Lookahead in Syntactic Error Repair, *ACM Trans. on Programming Languages and Systems*, 10(3):456–469.

Describes a property of a group of lookahead symbols which results in a reasonable error-repair algorithm.

Pai, A. B. and R. Kieburtz. 1980. Global Context Recovery: A New Strategy for Syntactic Error Recovery by Table-Driven Parsers, *ACM Trans. on Programming Languages and Systems*, 2(1):18–41.

This method uses fiducial symbols, not to do panic-mode recovery, but as the beginning of a set of legal tokens to be parsed; used in the context of LL(1) parser generators.

Richter, H. 1985. Noncorrecting Syntax Error Recovery, *ACM Trans. on Programming Languages and Systems*, 7(3):478–489.

Describes a recovery technique—so that compiler can continue finding errors—without attempting a correction to the error.

Waddle, V. E. 1990. Production Trees: A Compact Representation of Parsed Programs, *ACM Trans. on Programming Languages and Systems*, 12(1):61–83.

Introduces an Intermediate Representation more compact than abstract syntax trees.

EXERCISES

1. For the expression grammar

   ```
   E → E + T | T
   T → T * F | F
   F → (E) | Id
   ```

   find (a) FIRST (T), FIRST(T * Id) and (b) FOLLOW(E).

2. Show that the following grammar is not LL(1).

   ```
   A → d A
   A → d B
   A → f
   B → g
   ```

3. Show that the following grammar is not LL(1).

   ```
   S → X d
   X → C
   X → B a
   C → ε
   B → d
   ```

4. Write algorithms for computing FIRST and FOLLOW.

5. Rewrite the table in Example 4, as a programming procedure (using your favorite high-level language).

6. Given the grammar:

```
S  → XX
X  → xX
X  → y
```

   (a) Show that it is LL(1).
   (b) Create a parsing table.
   (c) Parse the string **xyxy**.
   (d) Draw the parse tree.

7. For the grammar

```
E  → T E'
E' → + T E' | ε
T  → F T'
T' → * F T' | ε
F  → Id | (E)
```

   (a) Show that FIRST(E) = {(, Id}.
   (b) Show that FOLLOW(T) = {+,) }.

8. Consider the grammar:

```
E  → E + T | T
T  → T * F | F
F  → (E) | ID
```

   (a) Left-recursion: Show what would happen if we tried to parse a * b + c using this grammar.
   (b) Eliminate the left-recursion from each production of this grammar to produce the grammar in Example 6.

9. (a) Show that the grammar

```
E  → E + E | E - E | E * E | E | E | (E) | Id
```

   is ambiguous (produces more than one parse for a given input).
   (b) Show that an ambiguous grammar cannot be LL(1).

10. The procedure for elimination of left-recursion need not be used if the grammar is not left-recursive. Write an algorithm that will test a grammar for left-recursion.

11. (a) Show that the assignment statement grammar of Chapters 1 and 2 has an indirect form of common prefix. The process of showing that it is not LL(1) will expose this.
    (b) Derive an algorithm for eliminating this problem.

12. Parsing non-LL(1) languages top-down anyway: It is sometimes possible to parse a non-LL(1) or even ambiguous language top-down by resolving the

choices at parse time. Consider the following grammar which abstracts IF-THEN-ELSE statements (i = IF, t = THEN, e = ELSE, a = terminal statement, c = condition):

```
S  →  i E t S
   |  i E t S e S
   |  a
E  →  c
```

(a) Show that this grammar is not LL(1).
(b) Create an LL(1) parsing table. (Since the grammar is not LL(1), there will be at least one double entry.)
(c) Show a top-down parse for

```
IF c THEN IF c THEN a ELSE a
```

associating "ELSE" with the closest IF, i.e., choose the table entry that will enforce this:

Stack	Input	Production
S	IF c THEN IF c THEN a ELSE a	

13. For the Ada subset grammar in Appendix B, compute the FIRST and FOLLOW sets for all the nonterminals.

PSOOL Compiler Project Part 2
Parser Generation

Use the grammar in Project Part 1, Chapter 3.

Option 1 (Easier)   Using a parser generator such as YACC (which generates a bottom-up parser described in Chapter 5), code the productions into the metalanguage of the tool and create a parser.

Option 2 (Harder)   Generate a top-down parser using the methods described in this chapter.

Run your parser on the programs (a) to (g) from Chapter 3.

5

Bottom-up Parser Generators

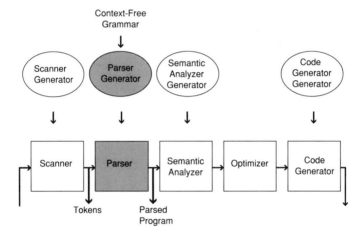

5.0 Introduction

Bottom-up parser generation follows the same form as that for top-down generation:

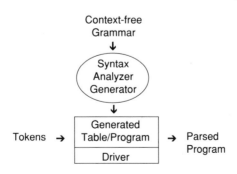

Figure 1

5.1 Metalanguage for Bottom-Up Parser Generation

The metalanguage for a bottom-up parser is not as restrictive as that for a top-down parser. Left-recursion is not a problem because the tree is built from the leaves up.

Strictly speaking, right-recursion, where the left-hand nonterminal is repeated at the end of the right-hand side, is not a problem. However, as we will see, the bottom-up parsing method described here pushes terminals and nonterminals on a stack until an appropriate right-hand side is found, and right-recursion can be somewhat inefficient in that many symbols must be pushed before a right-hand side is found.

EXAMPLE 1   BNF for bottom-up parsing

```
Program      →    Statements
Statements   →    Statement Statements | Statement
Statement    →    AsstStmt
AsstStmt     →    Identifier := Expression
Expression   →    Expression + Term | Expression-
                  Term | Term
Term         →    Term * Factor | Term / Factor |
                  Factor
Factor       →    (Expression ) | Identifier |
                  Literal
```

The BNF shown in Example 1 states that a program consists of a sequence of statements, each of which is an assignment statement with a right-hand side consisting of an arithmetic expression. This BNF is input to the parser generator to produce tables which are then accessed by the driver as the input is read.

EXAMPLE 2   Input to parser generator

```
Program      →    Statements
Statements   →    Statement Statements | Statement
Statement    →    AsstStmt ;
AsstStmt     →    Identifier := Expression
Expression   →    Expression + Term | Expression-
                  Term | Term
Term         →    Term * Factor | Term / Factor |
                  Factor
Factor       →    (Expression) | Identifier |
                  Literal
```

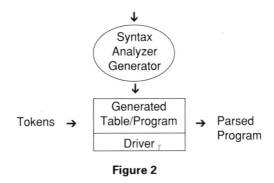

Figure 2

Using a context-free grammar, one can describe the structure of a program, that is, the function of the generated parser. The parser generator converts the BNF into tables. The form of the tables depends upon whether the generated parser is a top-down parser or a bottom-up parser. Top-down parsers are easy to generate; bottom-up parsers are more difficult to generate.

At compile-time, the driver reads input tokens, consults the table and creates a parse from the bottom-up.

We will describe the driver first, as usual. The method described here is a shift-reduce parsing method; that is, we parse by shifting input onto the stack until we have enough to recognize an appropriate right-hand side of a production. This is called the *handle*.

The handle is a right-hand side of a production, taking into account the rules of the grammar. For example, an expression would not use $a + b$ as the handle if the string were $a + b * c$. We will see that our method finds the correct handle.

5.2 LR-Family Parsing

The shift-reduce method to be described here is called LR-parsing. There are a number of variants (hence the use of the term LR-family), but they all use the same driver. They differ only in the generated table. The L in LR indicates that the string is parsed from left to right; the R indicates that the reverse of a right derivation is produced.

Given a grammar, we want to develop a deterministic bottom-up method for parsing legal strings described by the grammar. As in top-down parsing, we do this with a table and a driver which operates on the table.

5.2.1 LR-Family: Parser Driver

The driver reads the input and consults the table. The table has four different kinds of entries called *actions:*

Shift: Shift is indicated by the "S#" entries in the table where # is a new state. When we come to this entry in the table, we shift the current input symbol followed by the indicated new state onto the stack.

Reduce: Reduce is indicated by "R#" where # is the number of a production. The top of the stack contains the right-hand side of a production, the handle. Reduce by the indicated production, consult the GOTO part of the table to see the next state, and push the left-hand side of the production onto the stack followed by the new state.

Accept: Accept is indicated by the "Accept" entry in the table. When we come to this entry in the table, we accept the input string. Parsing is complete.

Error: The blank entries in the table indicate a syntax error. No action is defined.

Using these actions, the driver algorithm is:

Algorithm
LR Parser Driver

```
Initialize Stack to state 0
Append $ to end of input
While Action ≠ Accept And Action ≠ Error Do

Let Stack = s₀x₁s₁...xₘsₘ and remaining Input =
   aᵢaᵢ₊₁... $
   {s's are state numbers; x's are sequences of
   terminals and nonterminals}

Case Table[sₘ,aᵢ] is
   S#:   Action := Shift
   R#:   Action := Reduce
   Accept : Action := Accept
   Blank : Action := Error

EndWhile
```

EXAMPLE 3   LR parsing

Consider the following grammar, a subset of the assignment statement grammar:

```
1. E → E + T
2. E → T
3. T → T * F
4. T → F
5. F → (E)
6. F → Id
```

and consider the table to be built by magic for the moment:

State	Action						GOTO		
	id	+	*	(	)	$	E	T	F
0	S5			S4			1	2	3
1		S6				Accept			
2		R2	S7		R2	R2			
3		R4	R4		R4	R4			
4	S5			S4			8	2	3
5		R6	R6		R6	R6			
6	S5			S4				9	3
7	S5			S4					10
8		S6			S11				
9		R1	S7		R1	R1			
10		R3	R3		R3	R3			
11		R5	R5		R5	R5			

We will use this grammar and table to parse the input string, *a * (b + c)*, and to understand the meaning of the entries in the table:

Step (1)

Parsing begins with state 0 on the stack and the input terminated by "$":

Stack	Input	Action
0	a * (b + c) $	

Consulting the table, across from state 0 and under input **id**, is the action **S5** which means to **S**hift (push) the input onto the stack and go to state 5.

Step (2)

Stack	Input	Action
(1) 0	a * (b + c) $	S5
(2) 0 id 5	* (b + c) $	

The next step in the parse consults Table [*5, ** *]. The entry across from state **5** and under input *, is the action **R6** which means the right-hand side of production 6 is the handle to be reduced. We remove everything on the stack that includes the handle. Here, this is **id 5**. The stack now contains only **0**. Since the left-hand side of production 6 will be pushed on the stack, consult the GOTO part of the table across from state **0** (the exposed top state) and under **F** (the left-hand side of the production). The entry there is **3**. Thus, we push **F 3** onto the stack.

Step (3)

(2) 0 id 5	* (b + c) $	R6
(3) 0 F 3	* (b + c) $	

Now the top of the stack is state **3** and the current input is *. Consulting the entry at Table [*3*, *], the action indicated is R4, reduce using production 4. Thus, the right-hand side of production 4 is the handle on the stack. The algorithm says to pop the stack up to and including the F. That exposes state 0. Across from 0 and under the right-hand side of production 4 (the T) is state 2. We shift the T onto the stack followed by state 2.

Continuing,

(3) 0 F 3	* (b + c) $	R4
(4) 0 T 2	* (b + c) $	S7
0 T2 * 7	(b + c) $	S4
0T2 * 7(4	b + c) $	S5
0T2 * 7(4id 5	+ c) $	R6
0T2 * 7(4F3	+ c) $	R4
0T2 * 7(4T2	+ c) $	R2
0T2 * 7(4E8	+ c) $	S6
0T2 * 7(4E8 + 6	c $	S5
0T2 * 7(4E8 + 6 id 5	) $	R6
0T2 * 7(4E8 + 6F3	) $	R4
0T2 * 7(4E8 + 6T9	) $	R1
0T2 * 7(4E8	) $	S11
0T2 * 7(4E8) 11	$	R5
0T2 * 7F10	$	R3
0T2	$	R2
(19) 0E1	$	Accept

Step (19)

The parse is in state 1 looking at "$". The table indicates that this is the accept state. Parsing has thus completed successfully. By following the reduce actions in reverse, starting with **R2**, the last reduce action, and continuing until **R6** the first reduce action, a parse tree can be created. Exercise 1 asks the reader to draw this parse tree.

5.2.2   LR-Family: SLR(1) Table Generation

At any stage of the parse, we will have the following configuration:

Stack	**Input**
$s_0 x_1 s_1 \ldots x_m s_m$	$a_i a_{i+1} \ldots $ $

where the s's are states, the x's are sequences of terminals or nonterminals, and the a's are input symbols. This is somewhat like a finite-state machine where the state on top (the right here) of the stack contains the "accumulation of information" about the parse until this point. We just have to look at the top of the stack and the symbol coming in to know what to do.

We can construct such a finite-state machine from the productions in the grammar where each state is a set of Items.

We create the table using the grammar for expressions above. The reader is asked in Exercise 2 to extend this to recognize a sequence of assignment statements.

States

The LR table is created by considering different "states" of a parse. Each state consists of a description of similar parse states. These similar parse states are denoted by marked productions called *items*.

An item is a production with a *position marker*, e.g.,

  $E \rightarrow E \bullet +T$

which indicates the state of the parse where we have seen a string derivable from E and are looking for a string derivable from +T.

Items are grouped and each group becomes a state which represents a condition of the parse. We will state the algorithm and then show how it can be applied to the grammar of Example 3.

Algorithm
Constructing States via Item groups
  (0) Create a new nonterminal S' and a new production
      $S' \rightarrow S$ where S is the *Start* symbol.
  (1) IF S is the *Start* symbol, put $S' \rightarrow \bullet S$ into a
      Start State called *State 0*.
  (2) Closure: IF $A \rightarrow x \bullet X\alpha$ is in the state, THEN add X
      $\rightarrow \bullet \omega$ to the state for every production $X \rightarrow \omega$ in
      the grammar.
  (3) Look for an item of form $A \rightarrow x \bullet z\omega$ where z is a
      single terminal or nonterminal and build a new
      state from $A \rightarrow xz \bullet \omega$. (Include in the new state
      all items with $\bullet$ z in the original state.)
  (4) Continue until no new states can be created. (A
      state is new if it is not identical to an old
      state.)

EXAMPLE 4   Constructing items and states for the expression grammar

  Step 0   Create $E' \rightarrow E$

  Step 1
  State 0
  $E' \rightarrow \bullet E$

  Step 2
  $E \rightarrow \bullet E$ fits the model $A \rightarrow x \bullet X \omega$, with x, $\omega = \epsilon$, and X = E.
  $E \rightarrow T$ and $E \rightarrow E + T$ are productions whose left-hand sides
     are E; thus $E \rightarrow \bullet T$ and $E \rightarrow \bullet E + T$ are added to State 0.

  State 0
  $E' \rightarrow \bullet E$
  $E \rightarrow \bullet E + T$
  $E \rightarrow \bullet T$

Reapplying Step 2 to E → • T adds

```
T  →  •  T  *  F
T  →  •  F
```

and reapplying Step 2 to T → • F adds

```
F  →  •  (E)
F  →  •  Id
```

State 0 is thus:

State 0
```
E'  →  •  E
E   →  •  E  +  T
E   →  •  T
T   →  •  T  *  F
T   →  •  F
F   →  •  (E)
F   →  •  Id
```

If the dot is interpreted as separating the part of the string that has been parsed from the part yet to be parsed, State 0 indicates the state where we "expect" to see an E (an expression). Expecting to see an E is the same as expecting to see an E + T (the sum of two things), a T (a term), or a T * F (the product of two things) since all of these are possibilities for an E (an expression).

Using Step 3, there are two items in State 0 with an E after the dot. E' → • E fits the model A → x • zω with x and ω = ε, z = E. Thus, we build a new state, putting E'→ E • into it. Since E → • E + T also has E after •, we add E → E • + T. Step 2 doesn't apply, and we are finished with State 1.

State 1
```
E'  →  E  •
E   →  E  •  +  T
```

Interpreting the dot, •, as above, the first item here indicates that the entire expression has been parsed. When we create the table, this item will be used to create the "Accept" entry. (In fact, looking at the table above, it can be seen that "Accept" is an entry for State 1.) Similarly, the item E → E • + T indicates the state of a parse where an expression has been seen and we expect a "+ T". The string might be "*Id + Id*" where the first Id has been read, for example, or *Id * Id + Id * Id* where the first *Id * Id* has been read.

Continuing, the following states are created.

State 2	State 3	State 4	State 5	State 6
E → T •	T → F •	F → (• E)	F → Id •	E → E + • T
T → T • ⋆ F		E → • E + T		T → • T ⋆ F
		E → • T		T → • F
		T → • T ⋆ F		F → • (E)
		T → • F		F → • Id
		F → • (E)		
		F → • Id		

State 7	State 8	State 9	State 10	State 11
T → T ⋆ • F	F → (E •)	E → E + T •	T → T ⋆ F •	F → (E) •
F → • (E)	E → E • + T	T → T • ⋆ F		
F → • Id				

These are called *LR(0) items* because no lookahead was considered when creating them.

We could use these to build an LR(0) parsing table, but for this example, there will be multiply defined entries since the grammar is not LR(0) (see Exercise 10). These can also be considered SLR items and we will use them to build an SLR(1) table, using one symbol lookahead.

Algorithm
Construction of an SLR(1) Parsing Table

    (1) IF A → x • a ω is in state *m* for input symbol *a*, AND A → x a • ω is in state *n*, THEN enter *Sn* at Table[*m,a*].

    (2) IF A → ω • is in state *n*, THEN enter *Ri* at Table[*n,a*] WHERE *i* is the production *i*: A → ω and *a* is in FOLLOW(A).

    (3) IF S' → S • is in State *n*, THEN enter "Accept" at Table[*n*,$].

    (4) IF A → x • B ω is in State *m*, AND A → x B • ω is in State *n*, THEN enter *n* at Table[*m,B*].

EXAMPLE 5   Creating an SLR(1) table for the expression grammar

Following are some of the steps for creating the SLR(1) table shown in Example 4. One example is shown for each of the steps in the algorithm.

Step 1

E → E • + T is in State 1
E → E + • T is in State 6

so Table[1,+] = S6.

Step 2
In State 3 we have T → F •

The terminals that can *follow* T in any sentential form are +, *,), and $ (see Chapter 4).

So Table[3,+] = Table[3,*] = Table[3,)] = Table[3,$] = R4 where 4 is the number of production T → F.

Step 3
E' is the Start symbol here and E' → E • is in State 1, so Table[1,$] = "Accept"

Step 4
E → • E + T is in State 0, while E → E • + T is in State 1, so Table[0,E] = 1

5.2.3   Shift-Reduce Conflicts

If the grammar is not SLR(1), then there may be more than one entry in the table. If both a "shift" action and a "reduce" action occur in the same entry, and the parsing process consults that entry, then a *shift-reduce* conflict is said to occur (see Exercise 7). Briefly, a shift-reduce error occurs when the parser cannot decide whether to continue shifting or to reduce (using a different production rule).

Similarly, a *reduce-reduce* error occurs when the parser has to choose between more than one equally acceptable production.

One way to resolve such conflicts is to attempt to rewrite the grammar. Another method is to analyze the situation and decide, if possible, which action is the correct one. If neither of these steps solve the problem, then it is possible that the underlying language construct cannot be described using an SLR(1) grammar; a different method will have to be used.

5.2.4   LR-Family Members

In Section 5.2.2, LR(0) states were created: no lookahead was used to create them. We did, however, consider the next input symbol (one symbol lookahead) when creating the table (see SLR table construction algorithm). If no lookahead is used to create the table, then the parser would be called an LR(0) parser. Unfortunately, LR(0) parsers don't recognize the constructs one finds in typical programming languages. If we consider the next possible symbol for each of the items in a state, as well as for creating the table, we would have an LR(1) parser.

LR(1) tables for typical programming languages are massive. SLR(1) parsers recognize many, but not all, of the constructs in typical programming languages.

There is another type of parser which recognizes almost as many constructs as an LR(1) parser. This is called a LALR(1) parser and is constructed by first constructing the LR(1) items and states and then merging many of them. Whenever two states are the same except for the lookahead symbol, they are merged. The first *LA* stands for *Lookahead* since a lookahead token is added to the item.

It is important to note that the same driver is used to parse. It is the table generation that is different.

5.2.5   LR-Family: LR(1) Table Generation

An LR(1) item is an LR(0) item plus a set of lookahead characters.

$$E \rightarrow E \bullet + T, \ \{\$,+\}$$

indicates that we have seen an E, and are expecting a "+ T", which may then be followed by the end of string (indicated by $) or by a "+" (as in $a + a + a$).

The algorithm is the same as for creating LR(0) items except the closure step which now needs to be modified to include the lookahead character:

> Closure: IF A → x • X y, $\mathscr{L}$ is in the state, where $\mathscr{L}$ is the set of lookaheads, THEN add X → • z, FIRST(yℓ) for each ℓ in $\mathscr{L}$ to the state for every X → z.

We build the first two states here and leave the remaining (21) to the reader:

State 0: E' → • E , {$} where {$} indicates that the string is followed by $.

Applying the closure rule to this gives us initially E → • E + T, {$} as the next item here since FIRST (ϵ $) = {$}. Now, the closure operation must be applied to this and FIRST (+ T $) = {+}, so the next item is E → • E + T, {+, $}. The entire states 0 and 1 are:

State 0			*State 1*		
E'	→	• E, {$}	E'	→	E • , {$}
E	→	• E + T, {+, $}	E	→	E • + T, {+, $}
E	→	• T, {+, $}			
T	→	• T * F, {$, +, *}			
T	→	• F, {$, +, *}			
F	→	• Id, {$, +, *}			
F	→	• (E), {$, +, *}			

LALR(1) parsers parse fewer languages than do LR(1) parsers.

5.2.6   LR-Family: LALR(1) Table Generation

It is often the case that two states in an LR(1) state have the exact same items except for the lookahead. We can reduce the size of the ultimate table by merging these two states. There are ten pairs of states that can be merged in the items for Section 5.2.5 and Exercise 11. Two of them and their merged states are:

State i	*State j*	*State i-j*
E → E + • T, {+, $}	E → E + • T, {), +}	E → E + • T, {), +, $}
T → • T * F, {$, +, *}	T → • T * F, {), +, *}	T → • T * F, {), +, *, $}
T → • T * F, {$, +, *}	T → • T * F, {), +, *}	T → • T * F, {), +, *, $}
F → • Id, {$, +, *}	F → • Id, {), +, *}	F → • Id, {), +, *, $}
F → • (E), {$, +, *}	F → • (E), {), +, *}	F → • (E), {), +, *, $}

LALR(1) parsers parse fewer language than do LR(1) parsers.

5.3   Error Handling in LR-Family Parsing

As in LL(1) parsing, the driver discovers that something is wrong when a token which cannot be used in a reduction is pushed onto the stack. Error repair consists of adding or deleting tokens to restore the parse to a state where parsing may continue. Since this may involve skipping input, skipping to the next "fiducial" symbol (symbols that begin or end a construct, such as *begin, end, semicolon,* etc.) is often done.

5.3.1 Better Error Handling

It is possible to detect the error earlier than when it is pushed onto the stack. Error recovery algorithms can be more clever than those which replace symbols on the stack or in the input.

The literature describes many syntactic error handling algorithms. See the Related Reading section at the end of this chapter, especially Fischer and LeBlanc (1988) and Hammond and Rayward-Smith (1984).

5.3.2 Generator Errors

One particularly insidious error occurs when a syntax error is made in the BNF which is input to the parser generator. The message

    Error in Language,

which, although accurate, is not likely to inspire confidence in the end-user of the compiler of which the generated parser is a part.

5.4 Table Representation and Compaction

The tables for both top-down and bottom-up parsing may be quite large for typical programming languages.

Representation as a two-dimensional array, which would allow fast access, is impractical, spacewise, because the tables are sparse. Sparse array techniques or other efficient data structures are necessary.

5.5 YACC, A LALR(1) Bottom-Up Parser Generator

This section describes YACC, *Yet Another Compiler-Compiler*, written by Steve Johnson at Bell Telephone Laboratories in 1975 for the UNIX operating system. Like LEX, versions have been ported to other machines and other operating systems, and, like the discussion of LEX, the discussion here is not intended as a user manual for YACC.

YACC produces a parser which is a C program. This C program can be compiled and linked with other compiler modules, including the scanner generated by LEX or any other scanner. YACC can also produce RATFOR programs. Versions which have been ported to other operating systems can produce programs in other languages such as Pascal.

YACC accepts a BNF grammar as input. Each production may have an action associated with it.

5.5.1 YACC Metalanguage

The YACC metalanguage has a form similar to that for LEX:

```
Definitions     ← C declaration and token definitions
%%
Rules           ←          BNF plus associated actions
%%
User-Written Procedures              ←              In C
```

The Definitions section can contain the typical things found at the top of a C program: constant definitions, structure declarations, include statements, and user variable definitions. Tokens may also be defined here.

The Rules section contains the BNF. The left-hand side is separated from the right-hand side by a colon, ":". The actions may appear interspersed in the right-hand side; this means they will be executed when all the tokens or nonterminals to the action's left are shifted. If the action occurs after a production, it will be invoked when a reduction (of the right-hand side to the left-hand side of a production) is made.

Thus, a YACC input file looks like the following:

```
%{
#include1
#include2
#define ...
%}
%token ...
...
%%

Nonterminal : Right-hand side {semantic action 1}
            | Right-hand side {semantic action 2}
...
%%
C functions
```

Example 6 shows a YACC input file for the language consisting of sequences of assignment statements.

EXAMPLE 6   Sequences of assignment statements in YACC

```
%{
#include <stdio.h>
%}
%start program
%token Id
%token Lit
%%
```

```
Program :     Statements      {printf("Program \n");};
Statements : Statement        Statements {printf("Statements \n");};
           | Statement        {printf("Statements \n");};
Statement :   AsstStmt        {printf("Statement \n");};
AsstStmt :    Id ":=" Expression        {printf("AsstStmt \n");};
Expression : Expression "+" Term {printf("Expression \n");};
           | Expression "-" Term {printf("Expression \n");};
```

```
            | Term                    {printf("Expression \n");};
Term :        Term "*" Factor         {printf("Term \n");};
              | Term "/" Factor       {printf("Term \n");};
              | Factor                {printf("Term \n");};
Factor :      "(" Expression ")"      {printf("Factor \n");};
              | Id                    {printf("Factor \n");};
              | Lit                   {printf("Factor \n");};
%%
#include lex.yy.c
```

In Example 6, the lexical analyzer is the one output by LEX, or users may write their own (and call it "lex.yy.c"). Alternatively, a function called "yylex()", consisting of code to find tokens, could be written in either the definition section or the User-Written Procedures section.

YACC contains facilities for specifying precedence and associativity of operators and for specifying errors. An error production in YACC is of the form:

> B → error β {Action}

where β is an erroneous construct.

We will look at this example again in Chapter 6 when we discuss semantic analysis.

5.5.2   Functionality of YACC

The C code generated by YACC can be altered before compiling and executing. The generated parser "rules the show" in that it calls the function *yylex()* when it needs a token. Figure 3 shows a similar picture to that of LEX in Figure 2 of Chapter 3:

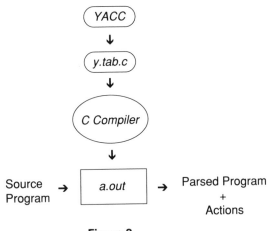

Figure 3

The metalanguage input is in a file called *translate.y*; the output of YACC is in a file called *y.tab.c.*

The input to the executable *a.out* program is again the source program because the *a.out* file contains the included scanner from LEX or the user-written scanner, *yylex( )*.

YACC produces a LALR(1) parser. The generated parser produces no output when presented with a correct source program unless the user-written actions contain output statements.

5.6 Summary

This chapter discusses parser generators, a much-researched and developed area of computer science.

The space occupied by the generated parse tables is considerable, containing thousands of entries. LL(1) tables are smaller than LALR(1), by a ratio of about two-to-one. LR(1) tables are too large to be practical.

Timewise, both LL(1) and LR-family parsers are linear for the average case (in the number of tokens processed).

It is easier to write a grammar for LR-family parsers than for LL(1) parsers since LL requires that there be no left-recursion or common prefixes. The LR-family grammars can also handle a wider range of language constructs; in fact the language constructs generated by LL(1) grammars are a proper subset of the LR(1) constructs. For the LR-family the language constructs recognized are:

```
LR(0) << SLR(1) < LALR(1) < LR(1)
LL(1) is almost a subset of LALR(1)
```

where << means much smaller and < means smaller.

The drivers for both LL(1) and LR-family parsers are easy to write. Table generation is easier for LL(1) than it is for LR-family parser generators.

Error handling is similar for both LL(1) and LR-family parsers, with LL(1) being somewhat simpler. Error handling in parser generators is still developing, and the Related Reading section contains many references to past and recent work in this area.

Overall, for parser generation the choice is between LALR(1) and LL(1), with the decision often being made based upon the nature of a grammar. If a grammar already exists and it is LL(1), then that is probably the method of choice. If the grammar is still to be written or the prewritten grammar is not LL(1), then the method of choice is probably LALR(1).

5.7 Related Reading

Aho, A., S. C. Johnson, and J. D. Ullman. 1975. Deterministic Parsing of Ambiguous Grammars, *CACM*, 18(8):441–452.

Burke, M. and G. A. Fisher. 1982. A Practical Method for Syntactic Error Diagnosis and Repair, *SIGPLAN Notices*, 17(6):67–78.

Cormack, G. V. 1989. An LR Substring Parser for Noncorrecting Syntax Error Recovery, in *Proceedings of SIGPLAN '89 Conference on Programming Language Design and Implementation*, Portland, OR, 161–169.

DeRemer, F. L. and T. Pennello. 1982. Efficient Computation of LALR(1) Look-Ahead Sets, *ACM Trans. on Programming Languages and Systems*, 4(4): 615–649.

Donahue, J. 1990. *Modula-3: A Case Study in Programming Language Design*, SIGPLAN '90 Advanced Topics Tutorial.

Discusses problems in language design, using Modula-3 as an example.

Fischer, C. N. and R. J. LeBlanc, Jr. 1988. *Crafting a Compiler*, Menlo Park, CA: Benjamin/ Cummings.

Contains an entire chapter on error handling for top-down and bottom-up parsers, as well as methods for table compaction.

Ganapathi, M. 1989. Semantic Predicates in Parser Generation, *Computer Languages*, 14(1).

Genillard, C. and A. Strohmeier. 1988. GRAMOL: A Grammar Description Language for Lexical and Syntactic Parsers, *SIGPLAN Notices*, 23(10):103–122.

Using Ada packages for implementation, and an unstratified metalanguage, scanners and either top-down or bottom-up parsers are produced, allowing for a dynamic change of source language.

Graham, S. L., C. B. Haley, and W. N. Joy. 1979. Practical LR Error Recovery, *SIGPLAN Notices*, 14(8):168–175.

Hammond, K. and V. J. Rayward-Smith. 1984. A Survey on Syntactic Error Recovery and Repair, *Computer Languages*, 9(1):51–67.

Harland, D. M. 1984. *Polymorphic Programming Languages, Design & Implementation*, London: Harland/Ellis Horwood.

Holub, A. 1990. *Compiler Design in C*, Englewood Cliffs, NJ: Prentice-Hall.

Contains a complete description, including a user manual and the C code for a top-down parser generator and a bottom-up parser generator.

Horspool, R. N. and M. Whitney. 1990. *Even Faster LR-Parsing*, 20(6):513–535.

Johnson, S. C. 1975. *Yacc—Yet Another Compiler Compiler*, C. S. Technical Report #32, Murray Hill, NJ: Bell Telephone Laboratories.

Probably the best-known, most often used compiler-compiler.

Mili, A. 1985. Towards a Theory of Forward Error Recovery, *IEEE Trans. on Software Engineering*, SE-11(8):735–748.

Mauney, J. and C. N. Fischer. 1988. Determining the Extent of Lookahead in Syntactic Error Repair, *ACM Trans. on Programming Languages and Systems*, 10(3):456–469.

Describes a property of a group of lookahead symbols which results in a reasonable error-repair algorithm.

Park, J. C. H., K. M. Choe, and C. H. Chang. 1985. A New Analysis of LALR Formalisms, *TOPLAS*, 7(1):159–175.

Richter, H. 1985. Noncorrecting Syntax Error Recovery, *ACM Trans. on Programming Languages and Systems*, 7(3):478–489.

Describes a recovery technique—so that the compiler can continue finding errors— without attempting a correction to the error.

Roberts, G. H. 1988. Recursive Ascent: An LR Analog to Recursive Descent, *SIGPLAN Notices*, 23(8):23–29.

Defines a procedure called recursive ascent which draws upon the closure operation in Item set creation.

Roberts, G. H. 1990. From Recursive Ascent to Recursive Descent: Via Compiler Optimizations, *SIGPLAN Notices*, 25(4).

A brief paper describing steps for conversion of LR parsers to LL parsers for languages that are basically LL.

Sager, T. 1986. A Short Proof of a Conjecture of DeRemer and Pennello, *ACM Trans. on Programming Languages and Systems*, 8(2):264–271.

A proof for language theory buffs concerning non-LR(k) grammars.

Snelting, G. 1990. How to Build LR Parsers Which Accept Incomplete Input, *SIGPLAN Notices*, 25(4):51–58.

Shows changes to shift-reduce actions which allow a reduction upon seeing a prefix of a sentential form. Useful for language-based editors and perhaps for distributed parsing (although the authors don't mention the latter).

Spector, D. 1988. Efficient Full LR(1) Parser Generation, *SIGPLAN Notices*, 23(12):143–150.

Stating that LR(1) grammars are more intuitive to write than LALR(1) grammars, the author argues further that minimal-state LR(1) parsing tables are not much larger than those for LALR(1).

Waddle, V. E. 1990. Production Trees: A Compact Representation of Parsed Programs, *ACM Trans. on Programming Languages and Systems*, 12(1):61–83.

Introduces an intermediate representation more compact than abstract syntax trees.

EXERCISES

1. Draw the parse tree for the string in Example 3.

2. Extend the table creation of Example 4 for sequences of assignment states. Parse the program:

```
X1 := a + bb * 12;
X2 := a/2 + bb * 12;
```

3. Right-Recursion: A right-recursive grammar, sometimes called tail-recursive, can cause an LR-family parser to be inefficient because too many symbols pile up on the stack before a reduction can be made.
   (a) Show an example of a right-recursive grammar that can be parsed by an SLR(1) parser.
   (b) Create an SLR(1) parser for your grammar, and parse a short string.
   (c) Develop an algorithm to eliminate right-recursion.
   (d) Use your algorithm on the grammar in (a) and the example in (b).

4. (a) Compute the rest of the LR(1) states for the expression grammar.
   (b) Create the LR(1) parsing table. Note that for items in state i of the form

$$A \rightarrow \omega \bullet, \ \{1_1, 1_2 \ldots\},$$

   $Table[i,1_1] = Table[i,1_2] = \ldots = R\#$ where # is the number of the production

$$A \rightarrow \omega.$$

   (c) Use the table to parse the string $Id * (Id * Id)$.

5. (a) Create the LALR(1) states for the expression grammar from the states in Exercise 4.
   (b) Create the table from the items in the states. Note the difference in size (since there are fewer states).
   (c) Parse the string $Id * (Id + Id)$

6. Write a driver algorithm:
   (a) Which uses an LR(1) table to parse
   (b) Which uses a LALR(1) table to parse

7. Parsing Ambiguous Grammars: Consider the ambiguous grammar of Exercise 12, Chapter 3 for IF-THEN-ELSE statements.
   (a) Augment the grammar with S" → S, and calculate the LR(0) items.
   (b) Create an SLR(1) parsing table. Is the grammar SLR(1)? Why or why not?
   (c) Parse the string "IF b THEN IF b THEN a ELSE a", resolving the ambiguity by associating ELSE with the closest IF.

8. Operator Precedence Parsing: For some grammars, precedence relations can be set up between the operators. Such grammars contain neither ε-productions nor two adjacent nonterminals.

   Most grammars are *not* operator precedence, but operator grammars can sometimes be written for small special purpose applications. Also, an easy way to improve an LL parser for a programming language is to parse the expressions using operator precedence.

   We will show this for the following grammar for arithmetic expressions:

   ```
   E → E + E
   E → E * E
   E → (E)
   E → a
   ```

   Since the precedence will be built into the table, we do not have to worry that this grammar is ambiguous.

   As usual, the table will be built magically for us to use (and then we will discuss how to build one in Exercise 9).

   The algorithm is simple:

	(	a	*	+	)	$
)			•>	•>	•>	•>
a			•>	•>	•>	•>
*	<•	<•	•>	•>	•>	•>
+	<•	<•	<•	•>	•>	•>
(	<•	<•	<•	<•	≐	
$	<•	<•	<•	<•		

   where $a <• b$ means a has lower precedence than b, $a ≐ b$ means a has the same precedence as b, and $a •> b$ means a has higher precedence than b. Thus for expressions, $+ <• *$, $(≐)$, and $* •> +$. We identify the handle by finding two symbols, a and b, such that a •> b.

Algorithm

Precedence Parsing

```
Insert precedence relations into input string,
with "$" 's at the beginning and end.
While Input ≠ $S$ DO
Scan to left-most •>.
Scan back to first <• to the left.
Reduce the handle that is between.
Reinsert precedence relations ignoring nonterminals.
EndWhile
```

Using the table and algorithm above, parse *(a + a)*.

9. Generating Precedence Tables: Because operators lower in the parse tree have higher precedence, we can build the precedence relations using these sets, called *leading* and *trailing* sets:

  Leading (N), where N is a nonterminal, is the set of all terminals that can be the left-most terminal in any sentential form derivable from N.

  Trailing (N), where N is a nonterminal, is the set of all terminals that can be the right-most terminal in a sentential form derivable from N.

  To generate the table:

Algorithm

Creating a Precedence Table

```
FOR each production of the form N → α A t B β,
Compute Leading(B)
Compute Trailing(A)
Use these sets to compute precedence relations:
```

t <• Leading (B)
Trailing (A) •> t

```
If terminals t₁ and t₂ appear on the right-hand side
                                of the production,
```

$$t_1 \doteq t_2$$

```
ENDFOR
```

(a) For the expression grammar,

```
1. E → E + T
2. E → T
3. T → T * F
4. T → F
5. F → (E)
6. F → Id
```

  compute leading and trailing for all nonterminals.

(b) Using the algorithm, build the table.

10. Show that the grammar for assignment statements (see the previous two chapters or Exercise 2) is not LR(0).

11. Finish the example from Section 5.2.5.

12. Finish the example from Section 5.2.6

13. Finish the finite state machine for the grammar of Example 4:

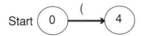

PSOOL Compiler Project Part 3
(Optional) Error Handling

Error handling involves four tasks:

(i) **Error Creation.** This is not a problem (there are more incorrect programs than correct ones in the world), although some language designs make it easier for the programmer to make errors. Ada is well designed in this respect; in Ada, comments do not go over line boundaries, a common error source.

(ii) **Error Detection.** Early detection finds the error, and as discussed in Section 5.3.1, both LL and LR parsers find the error as soon as it is pushed onto the stack.

(iii) **Error Reporting.** Good error messages are important. The offending token should be named, perhaps by pointing to it in the source program, and an indication given as to why it is wrong.

(iv) **Error Correction.** This is actually a misnomer, as it is only possible to correct the error by reading the creator's mind. Error *recovery* is perhaps a better word. At any rate, repairing the error may allow the parser to continue finding errors. It may also cause it to find spurious, nonexistent errors.

Consulting one or more of the references in the selected reading or the documentation for whatever tool you are using, or devising a method of your own, add syntactic error handling to your generated parser.

Run your error-handling parser on:

```
(a)
Action Wrong1
LocalNames xyz, b3, a, c, b, p : integer ;
Begun
  a := b3 ;
  xyz := a + b + c
    - p / q ;
  a = xyz * (p + q) ;
  p := a - xyz - p
EndAction ;
```

```
(b)
Action Wrong2
  BeginAction
LocalNames None
    If i > j Then ;
       i := i + j ;
    Elsif i < j Then ;
       i := 1 ;
    End of ;
  End ;
```

In (b), it is not a syntactic error that "None" is declared for "LocalNames". In fact, it may not be a semantic error if *i* and *j* are declared elsewhere.

```
(c)
Action Wrong3
  BeginAction
    While (i < j) and (j < k Loop
       k := k + 1 ;
       While (i = j) Loop ;

i := i + 2 ;
       End loop ;
  EndAction ;
```

Note that the *missing* "LocalNames" in (c) is a syntax error.

```
(d) An empty program
(e) Erroneous programs of your choice
```

6

Semantic Analysis and Attribute Grammars

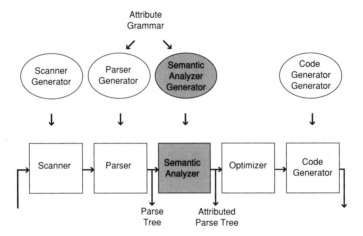

6.0 Introduction

The semantic analysis phase is a bridge between the parsing phase and the code generation phase. It includes such tasks as generating an intermediate representation (see PSOOL Compiler Project, Part 4, at the end of this chapter), creating a symbol table (see PSOOL Compiler Project, Part 5, at the end of this chapter), finishing the syntax analysis, and any of a myriad of tasks which prepares the program for the code generation phase.

A semantic analyzer generator does not follow the table/driver model developed in the previous chapters. The input, an attribute grammar, is more of a specification language than a true metalanguage.

In an attribute grammar, variables called *attributes* are attached to the nonterminals and sometimes the terminals of the grammar. These attribute variables can be passed to the parser generator, and at parse time, they can be added as tags to the nodes of the parse tree. The semantic functions in the attribute grammar describe how to give values to these attributes at parse time or after parse time.

Knuth (1968) developed attribute grammars as a formalism for the semantics of programming languages.

Most parser generators allow semantic actions to be attached to the productions in the BNF. A few allow these semantic actions to be described using attribute grammars. In this chapter, we will restrict our examples to attribute grammar descriptions.

With this chapter, we begin the study of compiler phases that may not be entirely generated. The amount of processing done at generation time depends on the attribute grammar itself. Consider the picture shown in Figure 1:

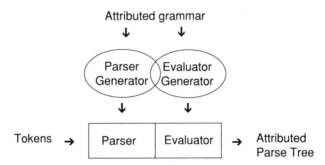

Figure 1 Semantic analyzer and generator

In some cases, the evaluator generator will be null, that is, an evaluator will not be generated. If the generator is null, it may be that the attributes were in a form that could be evaluated during parsing. Another possibility is that the attributes are evaluated after the parsing phase, but by a (hand-written) evaluator rather than a generated one. We will discuss all of these possibilities.

Attributes may be data types of variables and expressions, symbol table values, and even machine code for the statements in a program.

6.1 Metalanguage for Semantic Analysis Generation

The metalanguage for semantic analysis is an *attribute grammar*. An attribute grammar is an extension to a context-free grammar that allows a specification of semantics. It is also a formalism for expressing semantics much as a context-free grammar is a formalism for expressing syntax. In the next section we present some fundamental definitions that will be used later in the chapter.

6.1.1 Fundamental Definitions

An *attribute grammar* is a context-free grammar to which *attributes* and *semantic functions* have been added:

Consider a production p in the set of productions P:

$$p : X_0 \rightarrow X_1 X_2 X_3 \ldots X_n \qquad n \geq 1$$

For any X_i in the production p, there may be finite disjoint sets $I(X_i)$ and $S(X_i)$ called *inherited* attributes and *synthesized* attributes, respectively.

In general, the values of inherited attributes are passed *down* the parse tree. The values of synthesized attributes are passed *up* the parse tree.

The set of all attributes for X_i is denoted $A(X_i)$:

$$A(X_i) = I(X_i) \cup S(X_i)$$

An attribute a of X_i is denoted $X_i.a$ whether it is a reference to the grammar or to a parse tree. Below, we will distinguish whether the reference to attribute a is to the parse tree or the grammar.

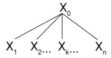

Predefined attribute values are called *intrinsic*. Synthesized, intrinsic attributes of terminals are computed by the lexical analysis phase. Inherited intrinsic attributes of the start symbol are passed as parameters before evaluation begins.

A production $p: X_0 \rightarrow X_1X_2X_3 \ldots X_n$ possesses an *attribute occurrence*, (a,k), if X_k has an attribute a, that is, $a \in A(X_k)$.

When a production $X_0 \rightarrow X_1X_2X_3 \ldots X_n$ is used in a parse tree at compile-time, where X_k is at node #m (in some tree-numbering scheme), then we say X_k possesses an *attribute realization* (a,m) if X_k has an attribute a. A *semantic function*, sometimes called an attribute rule, gives a value to an attribute occurrence (a,k) in production p. Such a function is denoted $f^p_{(a,k)}$.

The set of values upon which $f^p_{(a,k)}$ depends is called the *dependency set* for (a,k) and is denoted $D^p_{(a,k)}$. Thus,

$$D^p_{(a,k)} = \{ (b,j) \mid f^p_{(a,k)} = g(\ldots X_j.b, \ldots) \}$$

This is read "the value of attribute occurrence (a,k) or $X_k.a$ depends on the set of attributes $\{(b,j)\}$ or $\{X_j.b\}$ where each $X_j.b$ is used in the calculation of $X_k.a$".

Example 1 illustrates these definitions. This example is an adaptation from Knuth (1968) and is useful more to illustrate definitions than as an application of attribute grammars. We will see more compiler-oriented examples later.

EXAMPLE 1   The canonical attribute grammar example

Syntax	**Semantics**
0: Number → Sign List	(i) List.*Scale* := 0
	(ii) Number.*Value* := IF Sign.*Neg* THEN
	- List.*Value* ELSE List.*Value*
1: Sign → +	(i) Sign.*Neg* := False
2: Sign → -	(i) Sign.*Neg* := True
3: List → BinaryDigit	(i) BinaryDigit.*Scale* := List.*Scale*
	(ii) List.*Value* := BinaryDigit.*Value*
4: List$_0$ → List$_1$ BinaryDigit	(i) List$_1$.*Scale* := List$_0$.*Scale* + 1
	(ii) BinaryDigit.*Scale* := List$_0$.*Scale*
	(iii) List$_0$.*Value* := List$_1$.*Value* +
	BinaryDigit.*Value*
5: BinaryDigit → 0	(i) BinaryDigit.*Value* := 0
6: BinaryDigit → 1	(i) BinaryDigit.*Value* := $2^{\text{BinaryDigit.}Scale}$

The attributes in Example 1 are:

```
I(Number)       = φ
I(Sign)         = φ
I(List)         = {Scale}
I(BinaryDigit)  = {Scale}
S(Number)       = {Value}
S(Sign)         = {Neg}
S(List)         = {Value}
S(BinaryDigit)  = {Value}
```

Thus, *Scale* is an an inherited attribute, and *Value* and *Neg* are synthesized attributes. The intrinsic attributes are Sign.*Neg* in productions one and two, BinaryDigit.*Value* in production five, and List.*Scale* in production zero.

The function to compute $List_0$.*Value* in production four is denoted $f^4_{(Value,0)}$. Since $List_0$.*Value* depends on $List_1$.*Value* and BinaryDigit.*Value*,

$$D^4_{(Value,0)} = \{(Value,1),(Value,2)\}$$

Example 1 generates strings of binary digits. Example 2 shows an unevaluated parse tree for the string $- 1\ 0$:

EXAMPLE 2   Unevaluated tree

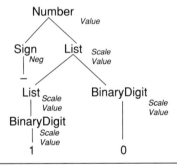

Section 6.2 discusses efficient methods for attribute evaluation, but we can "guess" at a method here: since we know *Value* is a synthesized attribute, and *Scale* is an inherited attribute, we can try to evaluate values by moving up the tree, then down, or by moving down the tree, then up. The latter suffices, and Example 3 shows the evaluated tree.

EXAMPLE 3   Evaluated tree

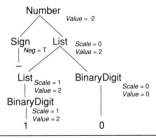

Example 3 shows that the "semantics" of this example computes the decimal value of the string and leaves this value at the root of the tree.

Examples 1 through 3 are a short and simple illustration of attribute grammars. It is possible to evaluate all the attributes in one pass down and then up the parse tree.

When a grammar is large and contains many attributes, it is not always easy to see how to evaluate the attributes. One method is to restrict the form of the attributes and attribute functions so that the method of evaluation is known. A second way is to create a graph of dependencies and check to see that it has no cycles. If it has no cycles, the dependency graph itself can be used to give an order in which to evaluate the attributes. We discuss all of these in the next sections.

Example 4 shows a simple but more compiler-oriented example. Attributes are used to pass information about the types of variables from where the information is known to where it is used in the tree. This information may then be used to enter values in the symbol table (see Section 6.3).

EXAMPLE 4   Assignment of types to variables

```
REAL     A,B,Q
INTEGER  X,Y,Q
```

The following BNF describes the syntax of these declarations:

```
Declaration      → Type List
List             → Variable
List₀            → List₁ , Variable
Type             → REAL | INTEGER
```

Adding an attribute called *Type,* not to be confused with the nonterminal, Type:

Declaration → Type List	(i)	List. *Type* = Type. *Type*	
List → Variable	(i)	Variable. *Type* = List. *Type*	
List₀ → List₁ , Variable	(i)	List₁. *Type* = List₀. *Type*	
	(ii)	Variable. *Type* = List₀. *Type*	
Type → **REAL** | **INTEGER**	(i)	Type. *Type* = **LexVal** (Type)	

The function **LexVal** returns the value found by the lexical analyzer (either REAL or INTEGER). Exercise 2 asks the reader to analyze this grammar.

Example 5 shows calculation of array offsets. This calculation might be performed in order to allocate the relative position of each array element.

EXAMPLE 5   Calculation of array offsets

```
List  → Id
List  → Id [EList]
EList → E
        | EList , E
```

where E is an expression. (We won't show the whole expression grammar here for simplicity. The reader has seen it enough!)

Consider the array reference:

```
A [I,J,K]
```

Suppose the array has been declared to have three dimensions and the range of the first dimension is d_1, the range of the second is d_2, and the range of the third is d_3. Then the offset is:

$$(I-1) \; * \; d_2 \; * \; d_3 \; + \; (J-1) \; * \; d_3 \; + \; (K-1)$$

Exercise 5 asks the reader to create attributes that will pass information about the array A (the dimensions d_1, d_2, d_3) down the tree and then to calculate this offset while reascending the tree. Exercise 6 asks the reader to consider a different grammar for this same example.

6.1.2   L-Attributed Attribute Grammars

A top-down parser can evaluate attributes as it parses if the attribute values can be computed in a top-down fashion. Such attribute grammars are termed *L-attributed*.

First, we introduce a new type of symbol called an *action* symbol. Action symbols appear in the grammar in any place a terminal or nonterminal may appear. They may also have their own attributes. They may, however, be pushed onto their own stack, called a semantic stack or attribute stack.

We illustrate action symbols using the notation "< >" which indicates that the symbol within the brackets is to be pushed onto the semantic stack when it appears at the top of the parse stack. By inserting this action in appropriate places, we will create a translator which converts from infix expressions to postfix expressions.

EXAMPLE 6   Converting from infix to postfix via an action symbol

```
E  →  TE'
E  →  T
E' →  + T E'  <+>
          | ε
T  →  F T'
T  →  F
T' →  * F T'  <*>
          | ε
F  →  (E)
          | Lit    <Lit>
          | Id     <Id>
```

We parse and translate $a + b * c$. The top is on the left for both stacks.

Parse Stack	Input	Semantic Stack
E $	a + b ⋆ c $	
T E' $	a + b ⋆ c $	
F E' $	a + b ⋆ c $	
a <a> E' $	a + b ⋆ c $	
E' $	+ b ⋆ c $	
E' $	+ b ⋆ c $	<a>
+ T E' <+> $	+ b ⋆ c $	<a>
T E' <+> $	b ⋆ c $	<a>
F T' E' <+> $	b ⋆ c $	<a>
b <b> T' E' <+> $	b ⋆ c $	<a>
T' E' <+> $	⋆ c $	<b> <a>
⋆ F T' <⋆> E' <+> $	⋆ c $	<b> <a>
F T' <⋆> E' <+> $	c $	<b> <a>
c <c> T' <⋆> E' <+> $	c $	<b> <a>
T' <⋆> E' <+> $	$	<c> <b> <a>
∈ <⋆> E' <+> $	$	<c> <b> <a>
<⋆> E' <+> $	$	<c> <b> <a>
E' <+> $	$	<⋆> <c> <b> <a>
∈ <+> $	$	<⋆> <c> <b> <a>
<+> $	$	<⋆> <c> <b> <a>
$	$	<+> <⋆> <c> <b> <a>

When the semantic stack is popped, the translated string is:

    a b c ⋆ +

the input string translated to postfix. In Example 6, the action symbol did not have any attached attributes.

The BNF in Example 6 is in LL(1) form. This is necessary for the top-down parse.

The formal definition of an L-attributed grammar is as follows. An attribute grammar is *L-attributed* if and only if for each production $X_0 \rightarrow X_1 X_2 \dots X_i \dots X_n$,

(1) $\{X_i.inh\} = f(\{X_j.inh\}, \{X_k.att\})$ $i, j \geq 1, \ 0 \leq k < i$

(2) $\{X_0.syn\} = f(\{X_0.inh\}, \{X_j.att\})$ $1 \leq j \leq n$

(3) $\{ActionSymbol.Syn\} = f(\{ActionSymbol.Inh\})$

(1) says that each *inherited* attribute of a symbol on the right-hand side depends only on inherited attributes of the right-hand side and arbitrary attributes of the symbols to the *left* of the given right-hand side symbol.

(2) says that each *synthesized* attribute of the left-hand-side symbol depends only on inherited attributes of that symbol and arbitrary attributes of right-hand-side symbols.

(3) says that the *synthesized* attributes of any action symbol depend only on the inherited attributes of the action symbol.

Conditions (1), (2) and (3) allow attributes to be evaluated in one left-to-right pass (see Exercise 2).

If the underlying grammar is LL(1), then an L-attributed grammar allows attributes to be evaluated while parsing. The reader may wish to review the LL(1) parsing driver in Chapter 4. The evaluation algorithm is:

Algorithm
LL(1) L-Attributed Evaluation

```
FOR each predicted production X₀ → X₁X₂...Xₙ.
  Push X₀'s inherited attributes onto semantic stack.
  Push X₁'s inherited attributes onto semantic stack.
  Parse X₁, then push X₁'s synthesized attributes onto
    semantic stack.
  Push X₂'s inherited attributes onto semantic stack.
  Parse X₂, then push X₂'s synthesized attributes onto
    semantic stack ...
  Push Xₙ's inherited attributes onto semantic stack.
  Parse Xₙ, then push Xₙ's synthesized attributes onto
    semantic stack.
  Pop attributes of X₁X₂,...,Xₙ.
  Push synthesized attributes of X₀.
ENDFOR
```

Exercise 3 asks the reader to combine this algorithm with the LL(1) driver algorithm given in Chapter 4.

Example 6 is LL(1) and L-attributed. Exercise 14 asks the reader to add actions to two versions of the expression grammar and compute the value of an expression without using action symbols.

6.1.3   S-Attributed Attribute Grammars

Attributes in an S-attributed grammar can be evaluated at parse time by a bottom-up parser. Interestingly, these grammars form a subset of the L-attributed grammars.

An attribute grammar is *S-attributed* if and only if:

- It is L-attributed.
- Nonterminals have only synthesized attributes.

This allows attributes to be evaluated during LR-parsing.

L-attributed and S-attributed grammars allow efficient evaluation—either during parsing or as a single pass after parsing.

In Section 6.2, we see another method and a different attribute restriction that allows attribute evaluation during top-down parsing.

For the next few sections, we focus on restrictions to attributes that allow for efficient attribute evaluation.

6.1.4   Noncircular Attribute Grammars

If the calculation of an attribute comes around to using its own value in the calculation, then we have a circularity. We will, however, need a more formal definition of circularity in terms of dependency graphs. We will also see in Chapter 8 that it is sometimes possible to evaluate attributes in a circular attribute grammar.

Dependency Graph of a Production

The dependency graph of a production, p, is a set of vertices and edges. The vertices are the attribute occurrences (see Section 6.1.1) and the edges are dependencies.

$$DG_p = (DV_p, DE_p)$$
$$\quad\quad\uparrow\quad\ \uparrow$$
$$\text{Attribute}\quad\text{Dependency Arcs}$$
$$\text{Occurrences}$$

Formally, for each production

$$p: X_o \rightarrow X_1\ X_2\ \ldots\ X_n,$$
$$DV_p = \{(a,k)\ |\ a\ is\ in\ A(X_k),\ 0 \leq k \leq n\}$$

and

$$DE_p = \{<(b,i),(a,k)>\ |\ (b,i)\ is\ in\ D^p_{(a,k)}\}$$

Thus, if O_1 is in the dependency set for O_2, then there is an arc between attribute occurrence O_1 and attribute occurrence O_2.

EXAMPLE 7   Dependency graph for a production

Consider production 4 from Example 1:

Production	**Semantics**
4. $List_0 \rightarrow List_1$ BinaryDigit	(i) $List_1.Scale := List_0.Scale + 1$
	(ii) $BinaryDigit.Scale := List_0.Scale$
	(iii) $List_0.Value := List_1.Value +$
	$BinaryDigit.Value$

DG₄:

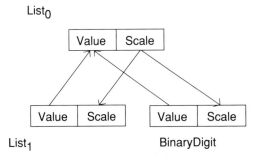

In Example 7,

$$DV_4 = \{(Value,0), (Scale,0), (Value,1), (Scale,1), (Value, 2), (Scale,2)\}$$
$$DE_4 = \{<(Value,1), (Value,0)>, <(Scale,0), (Scale,1)>, <(Value, 2),$$
$$(Value,0)>, <(Scale,0), (Scale,2)>\}$$

The dependency graph for an input program is produced by merging the dependency graphs for each production used to parse the program. It is defined in terms of the parse tree, T.

EXAMPLE 8   Dependency graph DG_T for input $-1\ 0$

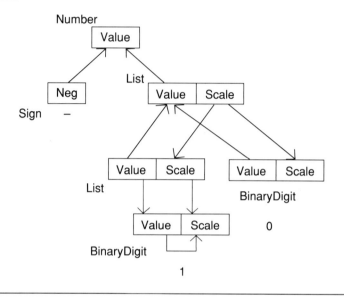

Since the dependency graph for an input is defined by augmenting the nodes of the parse tree with attributes, the definition of noncircularity is in terms of this parse tree:

An attribute grammar G is *noncircular* if there does not exist even one tree, T, such that DG_T contains a cycle.

Attribute grammars which are circular are undesirable. Knuth (1968, 1971) presents an algorithm which tests a grammar for noncircularity. It is exponential in the worst case. Jazayeri et al. (1975) show that there is no algorithm that tests a grammar for circularity which is not exponential in the worst case. Fortunately, most grammars do not exhibit this worst-case behavior.

6.1.5   Absolutely Noncircular Attribute Grammars

In Section 6.2 we present some efficient attribute evaluation methods. One of them requires that the attribute grammar be noncircular in an even stronger way than the noncircular definition above.

We start with the dependency graphs for the productions of a grammar. Figure 2 shows the nodes of the dependency graph for the binary digit grammar.

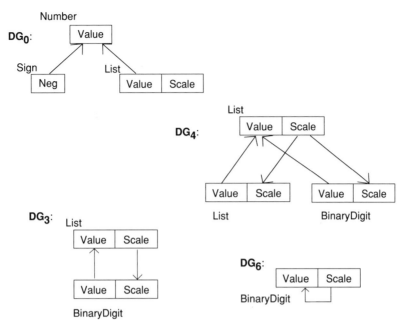

Figure 2   Dependency graphs

Example 8 shows these graphs merged to create the dependency graph for a parse tree, T. List's *Scale* attribute is handed down the tree to the BinaryDigit node where it is used to calculate the value of *Scale*. This value is handed back up the tree, changing as it goes, but ultimately it is used to calculate List's *Value* attribute. In functional notation, we would write:

```
List.Value = f(List.Scale)
```

where the function, f (the accumulation of the changes to *Scale* as it descends the tree), is used to compute *Value* and then is handed back up to the node. We indicate these closure steps by drawing an arc in the list node labeled with an asterisk, and we label the nodes themselves with asterisks, calling the new graphs *augmented dependency graphs*.

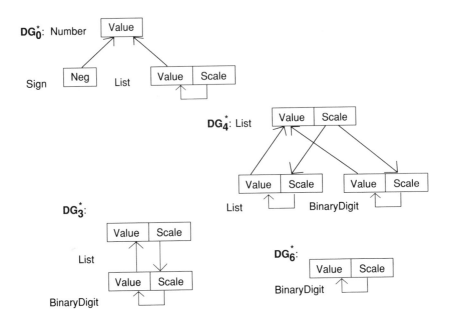

Figure 3   Augmented dependency graphs

With augmented dependency graphs defined, we can define *absolute noncircularity*. An attribute grammar is *absolutely noncircular* if none of the augmented dependency graphs, DG_p^*, contains a cycle.

Absolute noncircularity is a stronger restriction than noncircularity.

EXAMPLE 9   A noncircular attribute grammar that is not absolutely noncircular

$$
\begin{array}{llll}
S \rightarrow A & \text{(i)} & A.a = A.x \\
A_0 \rightarrow A_1 a & \text{(i)} & A_1.a = A_0.a \\
 & \text{(ii)} & A_1.b = A_1.y \\
 & \text{(iii)} & A_0.x = A_1.x \\
 & \text{(iv)} & A_0.y = 1 \\
A \rightarrow b & \text{(i)} & A.y = A.a \\
 & \text{(ii)} & A.x = 1 \\
A \rightarrow bb & \text{(i)} & A.x = A.b \\
 & \text{(ii)} & A.y = 1
\end{array}
$$

The augmented dependency graph for the first production contains a cycle (see Exercise 11).

6.2   Attribute Evaluation

Attributes are evaluated at compile-time on the parse tree. Even the dependency graph is a compile-time structure created from a parse tree; dependency graphs for the program are clearly not created at generation time. With restrictions on the grammar, such as absolute noncircularity, more preprocessing can be done at generation-time.

Evaluation methods which calculated attribute values during parsing were discussed in Section 6.1.

Before presenting some attribute evaluation methods, it is helpful to notice that *two* production must be used to evaluate attributes:

$$1) B \rightarrow \alpha X \beta$$

and

$$2) X \rightarrow \mu$$

The synthesized attributes of X are evaluated using the semantic functions corresponding to rule 2, but these can depend upon the inherited attributes of X, evaluated using semantic functions associated with rule 1.

In the same way, the inherited attributes of X are evaluated using those functions associated with rule 1, but it is possible that these depend upon other attributes whose values are calculated with functions associated with rule 2.

6.2.1 Vanilla-Flavored Evaluation

With no restrictions on the grammar, we can create a simple attribute evaluator that walks the parse tree evaluating attributes. A depth-first tree-walk is an easy algorithm to implement.

Algorithm

TreeWalkEvaluate (X_0) where $X_0 \rightarrow X_1 X_2 \ldots X_n$

```
WHILE there are attributes to be evaluated DO
  BEGIN
    Evaluate inherited attributes of X₀
    FOR i = 1 TO n DO
      TreeWalkEvaluate (Xᵢ)
    ENDFOR
    Evaluate synthesized attributes of X₀
  END
```

Little is done at compiler generation-time except to associate attributes and semantic functions with the productions.

Tree-walks tend to require gigantic storage requirements since most attribute grammars contain many rules which just move attribute values around. These are called *copy-rules*. They can be identified in a grammar as rules which just assign a right-hand side to a left-hand side. Also, calculation times for tree-walks tend to be long.

More efficient attribute evaluators can be created by methods which include dependency graph creation, grammatical restrictions, movement of some tasks to generation time, or some combination of these.

In the next section, we describe a number of ways to evaluate attributes more efficiently. With restrictions on the grammar, we can move some of the work back to evaluation time.

6.2.2   Efficient Attribute Evaluation: Use of Dependency Graphs

Section 6.1.4 describes dependency graphs for a parse tree, T. Creation of such graphs and their use to evaluate attributes is a way to improve upon evaluators that otherwise would make multiple passes over the tree.

The next section outlines a method presented in a paper by Kennedy and Ramanathan (1977). In this method, *some* of the processing is moved back to generation-time.

METHOD OF RAMANATHAN AND KENNEDY

The method outlined here, and described in further detail in Kennedy and Ramanathan (1977), generates a "semantic evaluator" which calculates attribute values using the dependency graph to calculate attribute evaluation order.

The dependency graph is, as usual, a compile-time structure, defined on the parse tree, not a generation-time structure.

The generated evaluator is called a "dynamic sequence evaluator" and, at compile-time, executes in three phases. We will describe these phases first and then move back to generation-time to see the tasks which can be performed to aid in the generation of this evaluator. The three compile-time phases are:

(1) Dependency graph construction

(2) Evaluation order creation

(3) Application of this evaluation order to evaluate attributes

DYNAMIC SEQUENCE EVALUATOR: (1) Dependency graph creation

The dependency graph described here will be augmented with instructions which will evaluate the attributes.

Suppose the nodes of the parse tree are numbered as follows:

   N(i) is the nonterminal at node **i**
   p(i) is the production used at node **i**

For example, if

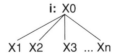

then,

$$p(i) : X_0 \rightarrow X_1 X_2 \ldots X_n, \text{ and } N(i) = X_0$$

To create the augmented dependency graph, it is helpful to distinguish the attributes in the grammar from those on the tree. In Section 6.1.1, we made this distinction by calling the former attribute *occurrences* and the latter attribute *realizations*. Example 10 shows these for a simple production.

EXAMPLE 10   Attribute occurrence vs. attribute realizations

$$p(5): \rightarrow X_1 X_2 \qquad X_1.a = X_0.a$$

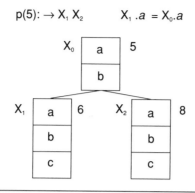

In Example 10, attribute a in the reference $X_1.a$ may be the attribute *occurrence* $(a,1)$ or the attribute *realization* $(a,6)$.

Also

$$N(6) = X_1 \text{ and } P(5) = X_0 \rightarrow X_1 X_2$$

One way to think of this is that attribute **realizations** correspond to *addresses* of attributes which are in the process of being evaluated. Attribute **occurrences** correspond to the formal parameters associated with the actual parameters (the attribute realizations) at evaluation time.

In this method, a semantic function is executed by a subprogram to evaluate $f^P_{(a,k)}$ whose dependency set is $D^P_{(a,k)}$.

The parameters to this subprogram are:

(a) An *operation code*: the code which implements the semantic function,

$$f^P_{(a,k)}$$

(b) The *output*: the realization (a,i_k) of (a,k) in $f^P_{(a,k)}$

(c) The *input*: the realization (a,i_k) of each (a,k) in $D^P_{(a,k)}$

EXAMPLE 11   From the binary digit grammar

```
4: List_0 → List_1 BinaryDigit    (i)   List_1.Scale := List_0.Scale + 1
                                  (ii)  BinaryDigit.Scale :=
                                                       List_0.Scale
                                  (iii) List_0.Value := List_1.Value +
                                                       BinaryDigit.Value
```

The subtree using 4:

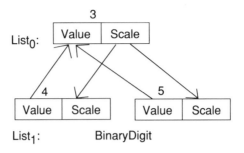

The instruction that corresponds to the third function (iii) has:

(a) Operation code: (4,3), the third function of production four.

(b) Output: (*Value*, 3).

(c) Input: (*Value*, 4) (*Value*, 5).

The instruction = (OpCode, Outputs, Inputs).

Such instructions will be executed by a "semantic function machine", SFM, much as we talk about the execution of Pascal programs as by a Pascal machine. First, we must associate these instructions with the dependency graph. Each vertex of the augmented dependency graph represents a unique attribute realization.

The vertex for the realization (a,i) is $V(a,i)$. Each vertex, $V(a,i)$, has an associated semantic instruction SI(V). Thus, SI($V(a,i)$) calculates an attribute a at tree node i.

Consider the tree and dependency graph in Figure 4.

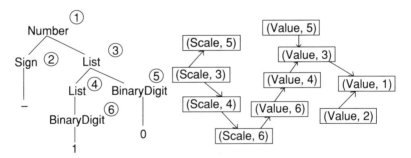

Figure 4 Tree and dependency graph for *−10*

The graph is constructed by walking the tree, visiting each node exactly once. The graph is a partial ordering of the attribute values.

The *Constructor* furnishes a "PLAN" which is executed upon visiting a node of the graph. There is one PLAN per Production. The PLAN which is executed upon a visit to node i is the PLAN associated with $p(i)$: $PLAN(p(i))$. We show Plan(p(3)) which is the plan for the production associated with node 3.

To execute PLAN(p(i)):

(1) For each $f_{(a,k)}^{p(i)}$, create $V(a,i_k)$ and add it to the graph.

(2) Create SI($V(a,i_k)$) by determining the realization of each attribute occurrence in $D_{(a,k)}^{p(i)}$.

(3) For each $f_{(a,k)}^{P(i)}$ and each (b,j) in $D_{(a,k)}^{P(i)}$, create an arc:

$$<V(b,i_j)\ ,V(a,i_k)>$$

For the tree and graph of Figure 4, three nodes are constructed after execution of PLAN(p(3)):

> (Scale,4) with instruction: ((4,1),(Scale,4),(Scale,3))
> (Scale,5) with instruction: ((4,2),(Scale,5),(Scale,3))
> (Value,3) with instruction: ((4,3), (Value,3),{(Value,4),(Value,5)}

Adding the arcs:

> $<V(Scale,3),V(Scale,4)>$,
> $<V(Scale,3),V(Scale,5)>$,
> $<V(Value,4),V(Value,3)>$,
> $<V(Value,5),V(Value,3)>$

This process is continued throughout the tree. The PLANS consist of high-level operations such as "find the nth child of node i". We have now finished (1) construction of the augmented dependency graph. Step two is:

DYNAMIC SEQUENCE EVALUATOR: (2) Determine the evaluation order.

(a) Use a topological sort of the dependency graph to produce a linear list:

$$(V_1,V_2,\ \ldots\ ,\ V_m)$$

The elements of $D_{(a,i)}^{P}$ cannot appear to the right of $f_{(a,i)}^{P}$.

(b) Create a straight line program of semantic functions:

$$(SI(V_1),SI(V_2),\ \ldots\ SI(V_m))$$

Step 3 is simple:

DYNAMIC SEQUENCE EVALUATOR: (3) Apply the evaluation order determined in (2) to the semantic function machine.

Remember that (1) encoded each attribute realization by address pairs. The evaluation order determined in (2) furnishes all the information needed to calculate attributes.

For each instruction, the semantic function machine calculates the addresses (on the tree) for the inputs and outputs and applies the code which executes the correct semantic function.

THE CONSTRUCTOR

The constructor has three tasks:

(1) A proof that the grammar is noncircular
(2) Generation of the semantic function machine
(3) Generation of the PLANS to construct the dependency graph

This is shown in Figure 5.

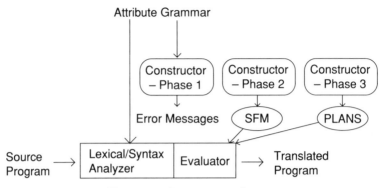

Figure 5 Constructor phases

CONSTRUCTOR Step 1: Since the circularity algorithm is exponential in the worst case, and its omission might cause the error, "Error in grammar", at compile-time, compromises are needed. Further restriction of the grammar is a possibility as is incomplete circularity testing.

CONSTRUCTOR Step 2: Generation of the SFM consists of (a) the code which associates the attribute realizations with attribute occurrences (independent of the grammar) and (b) generation of code sequences which implement each semantic function (grammar dependent).

EXAMPLE 12   Constructor, Step 2

$$(4,3): \text{List}_0.\textit{Value} := \text{List}_1.\textit{Value} + \text{BinaryDigit}.\textit{Value}$$
$$\downarrow \qquad\qquad \downarrow \qquad\qquad\qquad \downarrow$$

(a)   (R1)   (R2)   (R3)

```
(b)  MOVL       (R2),R0
     ADDL2      (R3),R0
     MOVL       R0,(R1)
```

Here, (a) associates the attribute realizations with the attribute occurrences, assigning the address of $\text{List}_0.\textit{Value}$ to R0, etc., and (b) shows the code sequence that implements the semantic function (4,3).

CONSTRUCTOR Step 3: Generation of a PLAN creates a series of instructions, many of which are independent of the language described by the attribute grammar. Procedures which create graph nodes and arcs are independent of the grammar itself.

COMPLEXITY

The complexity of the evaluator depends on the complexity of the semantic functions as well as on the number of nodes in the semantic tree. The formula is:

$$O\left(\sum_{i=1}^{|F|} m_i \left(T(f_i) + I(f_i)\right)\right)$$

where

$|F|$ = the number of semantic functions
m_i = the number of occurrences of each function f_i
$T(f_i)$ = the complexity of function f_i
$I(f_i)$ = the inputs to function f_i

For the constructor, the circularity test is exponential in the worst case and therefore dominates the complexity of the constructor.

METHOD OF KATAYAMA

In this method, nonterminals are considered to be functions which map their inherited attributes to their synthesized attributes. These functions are realized with procedures, and the method differs from tree-walk evaluators in that no information is attached to the parse trees except at the root.

The process begins by creating a procedure to compute the synthesized attributes of the start symbol. This procedure "calls" other procedures which must also be created. These procedures may be created at generation time.

More formally, let X be a nonterminal in an absolutely noncircular grammar G, and let s be a synthesized attribute of X. Associate with the pair (X,s) a procedure:

$$R_{X,s} (v_1, v_2, \ldots v_m, T; v)$$

where $v_1, v_2, \ldots v_m$ are input parameters corresponding to attributes needed to compute s, v is a parameter representing s, and T is a parse tree.

Procedure R evaluates the synthesized attribute s when supplied with the values of the input attributes and a parse tree.

Given a parse tree T_0 and a synthesized attribute s_0 of the start symbol S, we begin evaluation of s_0 by executing the procedure call statement:

$$\texttt{call } R_{S,s0} (T_0; v_0)$$

where v_0 is a variable corresponding to s_0.

To create a procedure $R_{X,s}$, examine the production used for the root node T and select a sequence of statements to calculate values of attribute occurrences of the production rule:

```
Procedure R_{X,s} (v_1, v_2, ..., v_m, T; v)
Begin
  Case production (T) Of
    p_1 : H_{p1,s}(v_1, v_2, ..., T; v)
    p_2 : H_{p2,s}(v_1, v_2, ..., T; v)
    ...
  Endcase
End
```

where

(1) "production(T)" is a function that returns the name of the production rule applied at the root of T,

(2) p1, p2, ... are production rules whose left-hand side is X, and

(3) Hp,s (v1, v2, ..., T;v) is a sequence of statements for evaluation of s when the production rule at the root of T is p.

To construct $H_{p,s}$, we perform four steps:

(1) For the production p: $X_0 \rightarrow X_1 X_2 \ldots X_{n_p}$, make an augmented dependency graph DG_p^*.

(2) From DG_p^*, remove nodes and edges not located on any path leading to $(s,0)$.

(3) To each attribute occurrence x in the attributes for X_0 which is not inherited, create an assignment statement for evaluating x. There are two cases:

> **Case 1**   If x is an inherited attribute of some X_k or x is s, then create the assignment statement:
>
> $$x := f_{p,x}(z_1, z_2, \ldots z_r)$$
>
> where $f_{p,x}$ is the semantic function for the attribute occurrence x and z_1, and $z_2, \ldots z_r$ are the elements of $f_{p,x}$'s dependency set.
>
> **Case 2**   If x is a synthesized attribute for some X_k, then create the procedure call:
>
> **Call** $RX_{k,s}$ ($w_1, w_2, \ldots, w_h, T[k]; x$)
>
> where $\{w_1, w_2, ..., w_h\} = \{(a, k) \mid x \text{ depends on } a\}$ and T[k] is the kth subtree of T.

(4) Let $x_1 x_2 \ldots x_m$ be attributes listed in a topological order on DG_p^*. Then the statements $H_{p,s}$ are listed in that order: the statements for x_1, followed by the statements for x_2, etc.

When x is S, the start symbol, and s is s_0, the procedure $RX_{k,s}$ is $R_{S,s0}$.

Procedure $R_{S,s0}$ may contain calls to other procedures $RX_{k,s}$, and they are constructed in the same way. Figure 6 shows an outline of the entire program.

```
Program KatayamaMethod
    Procedure R_{S,s0} (T;v);
    Begin
        ...
    End
    Procedure R_{X1,s1} (v_1,v_2, ...,v_m,T;v);
    Begin
        ...
    End
    ...
    Procedure R_{Xn,sn} (v_1,v_2, ...,v_m,T;v);
    Begin
        ...
    End
Begin {Main Program}
    Input parse tree T_0
    Call R_{S,s0} (T_0;v_0)
    Output v_0.
End
```

Figure 6 Outline of Katayama method

Example 13 shows this method applied to the Binary Digit grammar of Example 1 using the augmented dependency graphs from Figure 3. The example computes R_{List}(List.*Scale*, T; List.*Value*). By following the arrows in the augmented dependency graph, it is easily seen that for the nonterminals List and BinaryDigit,

> *Scale* → *Value*

This is why List.*Scale* is shown as an input parameter and List.*Value* is shown as the output parameter.

EXAMPLE 13   Computing R_{List}(List.Scale, T; List.Value)

Procedure R_{List} (List.*Scale*, T; List.*Value*)

Begin
  Case production (T) **Of**
    p_2: $H_{p2,\ Value}$ (List.*Scale*, T ; List.*Value*)
    p_3: $H_{p3,\ Value}$ (List.*Scale*, T ; List.*Value*)
  Endcase
End

Because the nodes of DG_4^* (except $List_0$.*Scale*) can be topologically ordered:

(1) BinaryDigit.*Scale*   (2) BinaryDigit.*Value*   (3) $List_1$.*Scale*
(4) $List_1$.*Value*   (5) $List_0$.*Value*,

$H_{p4,\ Value}$ is the sequence of statements:

```
BinaryDigit.Scale := List₀.Scale
Call RBinaryDigit(BinaryDigit.Scale, T[2];Binary-
Digit.Value)
List₁.Scale := List₀.Scale + 1
Call RList (List₁.Scale, T[1];List₁.Value)
List₀.Value := BinaryDigit.Value + List₁.Value
```

Figure 7 shows the entire program.

```
Program
Procedure  RNumber(T; Number.Value)
Begin
  List.Scale := 0
  call RList(List.Scale, T; List.Value)
  call RSign(T; Sign.Neg)
  Number.Value :=
    IF Sign.Neg THEN -List.Value
    ELSE List.Value
End

Procedure  RSign(T; Sign.Neg)
Begin
  Case production(T) Of
  p1: Sign.Neg := False
  p2: Sign.Neg := True
  Endcase
End

Procedure  RList(List.Scale,T; List.Value )
Begin
  Case production (T) Of
  p3: BinaryDigit.Scale := List.Scale
      Call RBinaryDigit(BinaryDigit.Scale,T; Binary-
                                              Digit.Value)
      List.Value := BinaryDigit.Value
  p4: BinaryDigit.Scale := List_0.Scale
      Call RBinaryDigit(BinaryDigit.Scale,T[2]; Binary-
                                              Digit.Value)
      List_1.Scale := List_0.Scale + 1
      Call RList(List_1.Scale,T[1]; List_1.Value)
      List_0.Value := BinaryDigit.Value + List_1.Value
  Endcase
End

Procedure  RBinaryDigit(BinaryDigit.Scale, T; Binary-
                                              Digit.Value)
  Begin
    Case production (T) Of
    p5: BinaryDigit.Value := 0
    p6: BinaryDigit.Value := 2 ** BinaryDigit.Scale,
    End
BEGIN {Main}
  Input derivation tree, T_0
  Call RNumber(T_0; Number.Value)
  Output(Number.Value)
END {Main}
```

Figure 7 Katayama's method for the binary digit grammar

6.3   Symbol Tables

The symbol table records information about each *symbol name* in a program. Historically, names were called symbols and hence we talk about a symbol table rather than a name table. In this chapter, the word symbol will mean *name*.

There may be more than one occurrence of a symbol name represented by the same identifier.

For example, a symbol may be redefined in block structured languages:

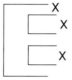

The picture implies that there is an outer block (or procedure) with a declaration of *x* and two inner blocks (or procedures) each with its own declaration of *x*; thus, the single identifier *x* again represents three different names or symbols.

Many compilers set up a table at lexical analysis time and fill in information about the symbol later during semantic analysis when more information about the variable is known. A classic example comes from the syntax used to refer to arrays and functions in FORTRAN and Ada. In both of these languages, *F(2)* might refer to an element F_2 of an array *F* or the value of function *F* computed using argument 2. For the lexical analyzer to make the distinction, some syntactic and semantic analysis must be added. Thus, such decisions are best postponed until semantic analysis time.

Symbol tables provide the following information:

- Given an identifier, which *name* is it?
- What information is to be associated with a name?
- How do we associate this information with a name?
- How do we access this information?

Some symbol tables also include the keywords in the same table. The alternative is to have a separate table for keywords.

6.3.1   Symbol Attributes

Each piece of information associated with a name is called an attribute (not to be confused with the term *semantic attribute*).

Attributes are language dependent, but might include the characters in the name, its type and even storage allocation information such as how many bytes the value will occupy.

The *class* of a name is an important attribute.

6.3.2   The Class and Related Attributes

A name in a program can represent a variable, a type, a constant, a parameter, a record, a record field, a procedure or function, an array, a label, or a file, to name just a few possibilities. These are values for an attribute called the symbol's *class*. Of course, not all languages have all of these possibilities (FORTRAN has no records) or they may be described using other terms (FORTRAN uses the word subroutine instead of procedure).

Once a name's class is known, the rest of the information may vary depending upon the value of class. For example, for a name whose class is variable, type, constant, parameter, or record field (to name a few), there is another attribute which records the names's *type*. Notice that this is somewhat recursive since *type* is also one of the possible classes. The recursion terminates with a name of some basic type. For example, in Pascal, the basic types are integer, real, character or Boolean.

For a name whose class is procedure or function, there are other attributes which indicate the *number of parameters*, the *parameters* themselves, and the *result type* for functions.

For a name whose class is array, other reasonable attributes are the *number of dimensions* and the *array bounds* (if known).

For a name whose class is file, other attributes might be the *record size*, the *record type* (sequential), etc.

Again, the possible classes for a name vary with the language, as do the other attributes (see Exercise 13).

6.3.3   Scope Attribute

Block structured languages allow declarations to be nested; a name can be redefined to be of a different class. A similar problem occurs when nested procedures or packages redefine a name. The name's *scope* is limited to the block or procedure in which it is defined. In Ada FOR-LOOP variables cause a new scope to be opened (containing only this variable).

Example 14 shows a main program with global variables *a* and *b,* a main program *Main*, a procedure *P* with parameter *x* and a local variable *a*. Information about each of these names is kept in the symbol table. References to *a*, *b*, and *x* are made in procedure *P* while main program *Main* makes references to procedure *P* and to its variable *a*.

EXAMPLE 14   Block structure

```
PROGRAM Main
   GLOBAL   a,b
   PROCEDURE  P(PARAMETER x)
      LOCAL  a
   BEGIN {P}
         ...a...
         ...b...
         ...x...
   END {P}
   BEGIN {Main}
      CALL P(a)
   END {Main}
```

The scope, perhaps represented by a number, is then an attribute for the name. An alternative technique is to have a separate symbol table for each scope.

6.3.4 Other Attributes

Section 6.3.2 describes how a name's other attributes may vary according to the value of its class attribute. Section 6.3.3 emphasizes the importance of a *scope* attribute.

Other attributes for names include the actual *characters* in the name's identifier, the *line number* in the source program where this name is declared and the *line numbers* where references occur.

6.3.5 Symbol Table Operations

There are two main operations on symbol tables: (1) *Insert* (or *Enter*) and (2) Lookup (or Retrieval).

Most languages require declaration of names. When the declaration is processed, the name is inserted into the symbol table. For languages not requiring declarations, such as FORTRAN, a name is inserted on its first occurrence in the program. Each subsequent use of a name causes a symbol table lookup operation.

Given the characters representing a name, searching finds the attributes associated with that name. The search time depends on the data structure used to represent the symbol table.

6.4 Implementing the Semantics of PSOOL Using an Attribute Grammar

The attributes we define here will be set-valued; their values will be sets (of Method Names).

Each attribute variable will be associated with a nonterminal or terminal of the grammar. Thus, in the BNF pseudocode for our example, the attribute variable *MethodList* (italics will be used for attributes) is associated with the nonterminal ClassDescription (as well as with various other nonterminals).

Consider, for example, the production defining the syntax of ClassDescription. To it (following the production) has been added a semantic equation defining a semantic value for a variable *MethodList* to be associated with the nonterminal ClassDescription.

At compile-time, the attribute *MethodList* will be evaluated at the node(s) ClassDescription:

```
ClassDescription      →
  Class            ClassName;
  SuperClass
         (SuperClassNames;|None;)
  InstanceVariables
     ({Inherit    InheritClassNames
     From ClassName;}⁺    | None;)
```

```
        Introduce  InstanceVariableDeclarations
                   | None;
    SharedVariables
        ({Inherit    SharedClassNames
        From ClassName;}⁺    | None;)
        Introduce   SharedVariableDeclarations
                   | None;
    Methods              (Methods| None);
    EndClass             ClassName;
```

$$ClassDescription.\textit{MethodList} := Methods.\textit{MethodList}$$

The attribute, *MethodList*, is associated with both the nonterminals ClassDescription and Methods. At compile-time, the value of *MethodList* is passed up the parse tree since the nonterminal Methods appears on the right-hand side of the equation and the nonterminal ClassDescription appears on the left-hand side, that is, *MethodList* is a synthesized attribute.

We show how inheritance, multiple inheritance, message passing, polymorphism, and even late-binding can be facilitated at compile-time by attribute grammars.

In what follows, we show separate parse trees for separate class declarations. In addition, it can be assumed that the parser can create a topological ordering in which to evaluate attributes. Thus, for our example, the attributes for *BankAccount* are evaluated before those for *SavingsAccount* and before those for *CheckingAccount*. The attributes for *SavingsAccount* and *CheckingAccount* are evaluated before those for *NOWAccount* and the attributes for all the class declarations are evaluated before those of the actions. This ordering is shown in Figure 8.

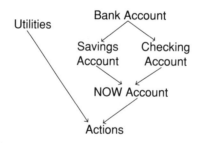

Figure 8   Attribute evaluation order

6.4.1   The Attributes

There are three attributes:

(1) *ClassName*, abbreviated *CN*, is an inherited attribute, passed down the class declaration tree to the Methods subtree. As the mnemonics imply, it carries the name of the current class down the tree.

(2) *SuperClassNames*, abbreviated *SN*, is an inherited attribute which descends to the Methods subtree and is used to make available the names of superclasses to the class.

(3) *MethodList*, abbreviated *ML*, is a synthesized attribute which, when it finally reaches the top of the tree, contains a list of methods available to the current class. Its value is a list of pairs: *ClassName* and *MethodName* for each *Method-Name* available to the *ClassName* and for each class name. They are ordered so that the methods belonging to the current class are listed first, with superclass methods listed second.

6.4.2 The Semantic Functions

The two productions of interest here are those for ClassDescription and Methods. The semantic functions follow each production.

```
ClassDescription      →
Class              ClassName;
SuperClass
              (SuperClassNames; | None;)
InstanceVariables
        ({Inherit    InheritClassNames
        From ClassName;}⁺    | None;)
        Introduce  InstanceVariableDeclarations
                    | None;
SharedVariables
        ({Inherit    SharedClassNames
        From ClassName;}⁺    | None;)
        Introduce  SharedVariableDeclarations
                    | None;
Methods            (Methods| None);
EndClass           ClassName;
```

(i)   Methods.*CN* = *LexValue*(ClassName)
(ii) Methods.*SN* = {*LexValue*
                    (SuperClassNames)}
(iii) ClassDescription.*ML* = Methods.*ML*

```
Methods  →
    ({Inherit          InheritMethodNames
      From ClassName;}⁺ | InheritNone;)
    Introduce (IntroMethodNames
                    | None);
    ({({Specialize SpecializeMethodName
      With MethodName Before;}⁺
        |{Specialize SpecializeMethodName
      With MethodName After;}⁺)}
                    | SpecializeNone);
    Definitions (Definitions
                    | None);
```

(iv) Methods.*ML* = Methods.CN &
        {*LexValue*(IntroduceMethodNames)}
      + Methods.*CN* & {*LexValue* (SpecializeMethodName'
                            NewMethodName)}

```
            + Methods.SN  &
            ({LexValue(InheritMethodNames)}
            - {LexValue (SpecializeMethodNames)})
```

where

  { } indicates an ordered list,

  & is defined for both elements and lists:
     a & {B, C, D, ...} is {a & B, a & C, a & D, ...}, and
     {a, b, ...} & {B, C, D, ...} is {a & B, a & C, a & D, ..., b & B, b & C, b & D, ...},
     where lowercase represents elements and uppercase represents sets,

  + appends two lists,

  − is set difference,
     {a, b, c} − {b} is {a, c}

a ' b appends the new method name b before or after a, according to the syntax.

6.4.3   Attribute Evaluation

Using a topological ordering, the attributes for *BankAccount* will be evaluated first,
then those for *SavingsAccount*, *CheckingAccount* and *NOWAccount*.

BankAccount

Attribute *CN* can be evaluated using function (i):

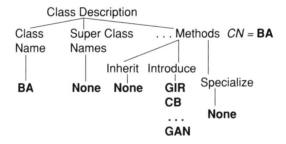

Attribute *SN* can be evaluated using function (ii):

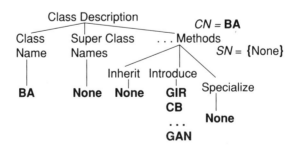

and *ML* can be calculated using functions (iii) and (iv). For function (iv),

Methods.ML = BA & { GIR, CB, ..., GAN } + None & ({None} − {None})
                + BA & {None}
                = { BA & GIR, BA & CB, ..., BA & GAN }:

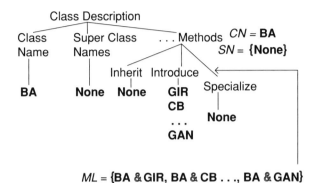

$$ML = \{BA\,\&\,GIR,\ BA\,\&\,CB\ ...,\ BA\,\&\,GAN\}$$

Function (iii) is simply a copy-rule and the completely attributed tree is:

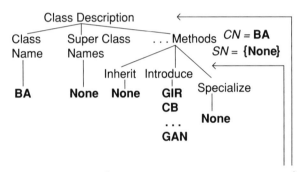

BankAccount $ML = \{BA\,\&\,GIR,\ BA\,\&\,CB\ ...,\ BA\,\&\,GAN\}$

The rest of the trees are shown after complete attribute evaluation:

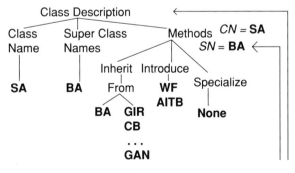

SavingsAccount $ML = \{SA\,\&\,WF,\ BA\,\&\,AITB,\ BA\,\&\,GIR$
                          $BA\,\&\,CB,\ ...,\ BA\,\&\,GAN\}$

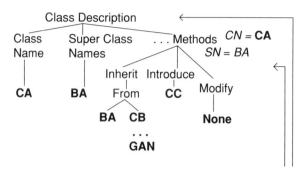

CheckingAccount   ML = {CA & CC, BA & CB, . . . , BA & GAN}

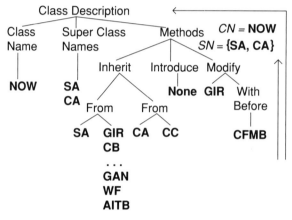

NOWAccount   ML = {NOW & GIR, SA & CB, . . . , SA & AITB,
                                     CA & CC}

The information left at the top of the trees can now be recorded in the symbol table, and when a message is sent within an *action*, the class of the receiving object can be checked for the validity of the selector as well as for where to find the corresponding method.

6.5 Summary

This chapter describes semantic analysis, the bridge between the front end and the back end of compiling. The specification of semantics is often done using attribute grammars, and much of this chapter has been devoted to attribute grammars. For this reason, the primary use of attributes, here, has been the automatic production of the front end of a compiler. The Related Reading mentions other applications of attribute grammars. Attributes are *evaluated* at compile-time; however, some processing toward generation of the evaluator may be moved back to compiler generation time.

Grammatical restrictions and efficient evaluation are interconnected in many cases. Thus, the attributes described by L-attributed attribute grammars can be evaluated at parse-time by a top-down parser or after the parse in a single pass down the tree.

The attributes described by S-attributed attribute grammars can be evaluated at parse-time by a bottom-up parser or after the parse by a single pass up the tree.

For unrestricted attribute grammars, tree-walk evaluators may require multiple passes over the parse tree.

More efficient evaluators may be obtained by creating a dependency graph from the parse tree and the semantic functions. A dependency graph ensures that the attributes upon which a semantic function depends are computed first.

The method of Kennedy and Warren (1976) uses a dependency graph, moving some of the operations back to generation time.

The method of Katayama (1984) moves much of the work back to generation time, but requires that the grammar be absolutely non-circular.

In Chapter 8, we will see attributes used to perform a high-level (on the parse tree) data flow analysis. The method of evaluation, as well as the attributes and semantic functions themselves, will be quite different from the methods described in this chapter. In Chapter 11, we will discuss attribute evaluation again when we discuss incremental compilation.

Another task of semantic analysis is symbol table creation. Symbol tables may be created by using attribute grammars; an attribute representing information about a name is moved around the tree until it reaches the name much as in Example 4. Name nodes can contain pointers to their entry in the symbol table.

Yet another task of semantic analysis is creation of an intermediate representation of the program. Part 4 of the PSOOL Compiler Project describes one form: an abstract syntax tree (AST). Chapter 7 discusses others: quadruples and DAG's.

6.6   Related Reading

Babich, W. A. and M. Jazayeri. 1978. The Methods of Attributes for Data Flow Analysis, Part I. Exhaustive Analysis, *Acta Informatica,* 10:245–264.

Contains a sample attribute grammar for performing data flow analysis on a tree.

Babich, W. A. and M. Jazayeri. 1978. The Methods of Attributes for Data Flow Analysis, Part II. Demand Analysis, *Acta Informatica,* 10:265–272.

Same as the preceding except the data flow information is computed when needed by the optimizer.

Bochmann, G. V. and P. Ward. 1978. Compiler Writing System for Attribute Grammars, *Computer Journal,* 21(2):144–148.

Bryant, B. R., E. Belanjaninath, S. Hull. 1986. Two-Level Grammars as an Implementable Metalanguage for Axiomatic Semantics, *Computer Languages,* 11(3/4).

Chapman, N. 1989. Regular Attribute Grammars and Finite State Machines, *SIGPLAN Notices,* 24(6):97–104.

Using an attribute grammar whose underlying context-free-grammar is regular (right or left linear), restricts attribute dependencies, and allows for efficient attribute evaluation. Since most programming language grammars are not regular, the applications are primarily for those which add semantics to the scanning process.

Courcelle, B. and P. Franchi-Zannettacci. 1982. Attribute Grammars and Recursive Program Schemes, *TCS,* 17(1 & 2).

Demers, A., T. Reps, and T. Teitelbaum. *Attribute Propagation by Message Passing,* ACM SIGPLAN 85 Symposium on Language Issues in Programming Environments.

Deransart, P., M. Jourdan, and B. Lorho. 1988. *Attribute Grammars: Definitions, Systems, Bibliography,* LNCS 323, Berlin: Springer-Verlag.

Dobler, H. and K. Pirklbauer. 1990. Coco-2, A New Compiler Compiler, *SIGPLAN Notices,* 25(5):82–90.

> *Uses separate metalanguages for scanner generation and parser/evaluator generation, but within the same file, producing a Modula-2 scanner and top-down parser with inherited and synthesized attribute evaluation via Modula-2 parameters and procedures.*

Farrow, R. 1982. Experience with an Attribute Grammar-Based Compiler, Ninth ACM Symposium on Principles of Programming Languages, 95–107.

Hammond, K. and V. J. Rayward-Smith. 1984. A Survey on Syntactic Error Recovery and Repair, *Computer Languages,* 9(7):51–67

Jazayeri, M., W. Ogden, and W. Rounds. 1975. The Intrinsic Exponential Complexity of the Circularity Problem for Attribute Grammars, *CACM,* 18(12):697–706.

Jones, L. G. 1990. Efficient Evaluation of Circular Attribute Grammars, *Trans. on Programming Languages and Systems,* 12(3):429–462.

Katayama, T. 1984. Translation of Attribute Grammars into Procedures, *ACM Trans. on Programming Languages and Systems,* 6(3).

> *The recursive descent of attribute grammars. A procedure is created for each nonterminal to which an attribute is attached and calls made to other procedures to perform the evaluation.*

Kennedy, K. and S. K. Warren, 1976. Automatic Generation of Efficient Evaluators for Attribute Grammars, Third ACM Symposium on Principles of Programming Languages, 32–49.

> *Describes a method which which creates an attribute evaluator (for absolutely non-circular attribute grammars) at compiler generation time*

Kennedy, K. and J. Ramanathan, 1977. *A Deterministic Attribute Grammar Evaluator Based on Dynamic Sequencing,* Fourth ACM Symposium on Principles of Programming Languages, 72–85.

> *While some of the work is facilitated at compiler generation time, the evaluator itself is created at compile-time.*

Knuth, D. E. 1968. Semantics of Context-Free Languages, *Mathematical Systems Theory,* 2(2):127–45.

> *The seminal article on attribute grammars.*

Knuth, D. E. 1971. Semantics of Context-Free Languages: Correction, *Mathematical Systems Theory,* 5(1):95.

> *Provides a correction to the proof that all inherited attributes can be mapped to synthesized attributes.*

Lemone, K. A. 1990. Document Formatting Using Attribute Grammars, WPI Technical Report Series, 2, Worcester, MA: Worcester Polytechnic Institute.

Lemone, K. A., J. McConnell, M. O'Connor, and J. Wisniewski. 1991. Implementing Semantics of Object-Oriented Languages Using Attribute Grammars, in Proceedings of the ACM 19th Computer Science Conference, San Antonio, TX.

Lorho, B., Ed. 1984. *Methods and Tools for Compiler Construction*, London: Cambridge University Press.

A collection of articles covering the compilation process with some emphasis on attribute grammars. The authors are well known for the area about which they write.

Meek, B. 1990. The Static Semantics File, *SIGPLAN Notices*, 25(4):33–42.

If you think you know what static semantics is, you may find your "knowledge" challenged in this series of EMail messages.

Noonan, R. E. *An Algorithm for Generating Abstract Syntax Trees,* 10(3/4):225–236.

O'Connor, M. and K. A. Lemone, 1987. *A Method to Improve Testing and Debugging of Robotic Programs in the Language Development Environment*, Proceedings of the ACM Computer Science Conference, St. Louis.

Uses attribute grammars to perform incremental editing of robotic programs.

Sonnenschein, M. 1987. Graph Translation Schemes to Generate Compiler Parts, *ACM Trans. on Programming Languages and Systems*, 9(4):473–490.

Modifies traditional attribute grammars to deal with program graphs and with conditional and iterative evaluation of attributes.

EXERCISES

1. (a) Calculate the values of the attributes *Scale* and *Value* for the parse tree as shown in Example 3 using the grammar from Example 1.
   (b) Parse and evaluate attributes for the string + *1001* using the grammar from Example 1.

2. For the attribute grammar of Example 4:
   (a) Is the attribute *Type* inherited or synthesized?
   (b) Is the grammar L-attributed? S-attributed?
   (c) Show that the grammar is noncircular.
   (d) Show that the grammar is absolutely noncircular.
   (e) Create a dependency graph for **REAL A, B, Q**.

3. (a) Show that the attributes in an L-attributed grammar can be evaluated in one left-to-right pass.
   (b) Show that the attributes in an L-attributed grammar can be evaluated by a top-down parser (whose underlying grammar is LL(1)).

4. Combine the LL(1)-attributed evaluation algorithm with the LL(1) driver algorithm from Chapter 4.

5. Find a way to evaluate attributes of an L-attributed grammar when the underlying grammar is not LL(1).

6. Consider the grammar of Example 5:
   (a) Create an inherited attribute called *Dims* which fetches the values d_1, d_2, and d_3 from the symbol table at node A and then passes these three values down the tree.

(b) Create synthesized attributes *NDim* and *Offset* that compute the number of dimensions in an array reference (as an error check) and compute the array offset, respectively, while climbing the tree.

7. If we change the grammar of Example 5 and Exercise 6, we can calculate both *NDim* and *Offset* in one pass up the tree. The original grammar results in the following tree:

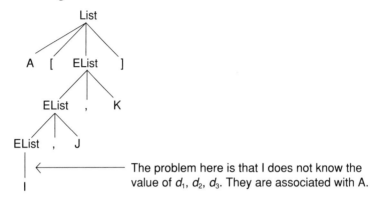

The problem here is that I does not know the value of d_1, d_2, d_3. They are associated with A.

In Exercise 6, we transmitted the values d_1, d_2 and d_3 down the tree to I to begin the calculation of the offset and ascended the tree, calculating the *Offset* and the value of *NDim*.

If we change the grammar to:

```
List  →  EList]
List  →  Id
EList → EList, E
EList → Id [ E
```

and attach semantic functions to calculate *Offset* and *NDim*, then we can calculate the values in one pass up the tree:

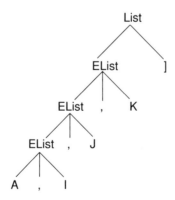

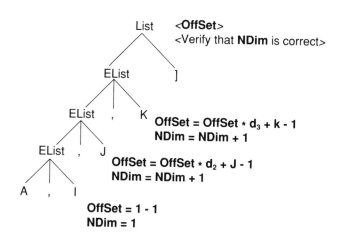

(a) Write the semantic functions which result in the above calculations.

(b) Show that your grammar is or is not L-attributed.

(c) Show that your grammar is or is not S-attributed.

8. Describe some grammar-independent procedures which a PLAN generator (as described in Section 6.2 in the method of Ramanathan and Kennedy) might create.

9. Write a *translation* grammar which will convert octal numbers to binary. (Hint: the BNF generates the octal numbers.)

10. Consider the following attributed grammar for a program consisting of a single assignment statement. The minus sign, −, in (iv) and (v) of production 3 represents set difference.

Productions

```
1. Program → BEGIN  Statement  END
2. Statement → Assignment



3. Assignment → Variable := Expression
```

Semantics

```
(i)   Statement.Live := Statement.Use
(i)   Statement.Use := Assignment.Use
(ii)  Statement.Defn := Assignment.Defn
(iii) Assignment.Live := Statement.Live
(i)   Expression.Use := {Variables in
                                 Expression}
(ii)  Variable.Defn := {LexValue
                                 (Variable)}
(iii) Assignment.Defn := Variable.Defn
(iv)  Assignment.Use := Expression.Use -
                            Variable.Defn
(v)   Variable.Live := Assignment. Live -
                            Variable.Live
(vi)  Expression.Live := Expression.Use
```

Expression can be any valid expression, e.g., $A + B$.

(a) List the synthesized and inherited attributes.

(b) Parse and evaluate attributes for the program:

```
BEGIN
  B := A + B
END
```

11. Write an attributed translation grammar using the BNF in Exercise 10 which will create an abstract syntax tree such as

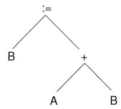

12. Show that the grammar of Example 9 is noncircular, but not absolutely noncircular.

13. Consider your favorite high-level language and design symbol table categories for its names.

14. (a) Using the following grammar for expressions, create a synthesized attribute *Value* and semantic functions which leave the calculated value of an expression at the top of a parse tree. Show that your grammar is S-attributed.

$$E \rightarrow E + T$$
$$E \rightarrow T$$
$$T \rightarrow T * F$$
$$T \rightarrow F$$
$$F \rightarrow (E)$$
$$F \rightarrow \textbf{Const}$$

(b) Using the following grammar for expressions, create a synthesized attribute *Value* and semantic functions which leave the calculated value of an expression at the top of a parse tree. Show that your grammar is L-attributed.

$$E \rightarrow TE'$$
$$E_0 \rightarrow + TE_1'$$
$$E' \rightarrow \epsilon$$
$$T \rightarrow FT'$$
$$T_0' \rightarrow * F T_1'$$
$$T' \rightarrow \epsilon$$
$$F \rightarrow (E)$$
$$F \rightarrow \textbf{Const}$$

15. Consider the following attribute grammar:

BNF	Semantic Functions
$N_1 \rightarrow N_2$ **c**	$N_1.CNum = N_2.CNum + 1$
	$N_1.DNum = N_2.DNum$
$N_1 \rightarrow N_2$ **d**	$N_1.CNum = N_2.CNum$
	$N_1.DNum = N_2.DNum + 1$
$N \rightarrow$ **d**	$N.CNum = 0$
	$N.DNum = 1$
$N \rightarrow$ **c**	$N.CNum = 1$
	$N.DNum = 0$

(a) Show that the grammar is or is not L-attributed.
(b) Show that the underlying grammar is or is not LL(1).
(c) Show that the grammar is or is not S-attributed
(d) Show that the underlying grammar is or is not LR(1).

16. The following grammar computes the same attribute as does the grammar of Example 1. Add the semantic functions for the first two productions to accomplish this.

```
1. N             → . List            N.Value = ...
2. List0         → BinaryDigit List  List.Value = ...
3. List          → BinaryDigit       List.Value =
                                          Binary Digit.Value
4. BinaryDigit → 0                   BinaryDigit.Value = 0
5. BinaryDigit → 1                   BinaryDigit.Value = 0.5
```

PSOOL Compiler Project Parts 4–6

There is no project assigned for Chapters 7 to 9, and the project parts described here should extend over several weeks, while the materials in this chapter and the next few are being read.

PSOOL Compiler Project Part 4
Abstract Syntax Trees

Average Time: 25–30 hours
For the statements in PSOOL, write attributes and semantic functions which will translate statements to abstract syntax trees.

Abstract Syntax Trees

Abstract syntax trees are an intermediate representation more suitable for optimization and code generation than parse trees. For this part of the project, you are to define a set of abstract syntax tree nodes for the language which your compiler currently implements. Add attributes and semantic functions to perform this translation:

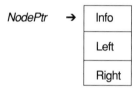

```
         plus
        /    \
     opnd₁  opnd₂
```

is an AST node for $a + b$ where a is opnd$_1$ and b is opnd$_2$.
   In parenthesized form, this could be written:

```
(plus ("a" "b"))  or  (+ ("a" "b"))
```

Two of the productions that relate to such a node are:

```
...
Relation              → SimpleExpression
SimpleExpression  → Term₁ {AddingOperator Term₂}
...
```

(The dots represent the productions which come before and after these two.)
   If we create a data structure for the nodes of the abstract syntax tree:

$$NodePtr \quad \rightarrow \quad \boxed{\begin{array}{c} \text{Info} \\ \hline \text{Left} \\ \hline \text{Right} \end{array}}$$

then we can add attributes such as the following:

```
...
Relation              → SimpleExpression
                            Relation.NodePtr = SimpleExpression.NodePtr
SimpleExpression  → Term₁ {AddingOperator Term₂}
                            SimpleExpression.NodePtr := {GetNode}
                            SimpleExpression.Info  := "+"
                            SimpleExpression.Left  := Term₁.NodePtr
                            SimpleExpression.Right := Term₂.NodePtr
```

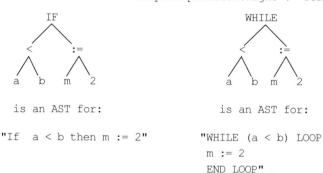

```
        IF                                  WHILE
       /  \                                /    \
      <    :=                             <      :=
     / \   / \                           / \    / \
    a   b m   2                         a   b  m   2

  is an AST for:                       is an AST for:

"If  a < b then m := 2"               "WHILE (a < b) LOOP
                                        m := 2
                                       END LOOP"
```

In parenthesized form these might be written:

```
(IF ("<" ("a" "b") ":=" ("m" "2"))) and
(WHILE ("<" ("a" "b") ":=" ("m" "2")))
```

or, with some indenting,

```
(IF
  ( "<" ("a" "b")
  ":=" ("m" "2"))) and
(WHILE
  ("<" ("a" "b")
  ":=" ("m" "2")))
```

(Other indentings are possible here.)

Attributes and semantic functions may be added analogously to those of the "+" node above. Design attributes and semantic functions which will translate your programs to abstract syntax trees.

Add semantic actions to whatever tool you are using to translate input programs to AST's.

Print them out in parenthesized form. The following is sample output of the first program (from the project description of Chapter 3):

```
Unit [
  Line(1)
  (Action (One)
  Line(2)
  (IntTypes
     (a b c xyz p q))
  Line(3)
  (BeginAction)
  Line(4)
  (:=
     (a, b3))
  (:=
  Line(5-6)
  (xyz, +
            (a +
               (b -
                  (c /
                     (p q))))))
  Line(7)
  (:=
        (a *
           (xyz +
               (p q))))
  Line(8)
  (:=
     (p -
        (a  -
           (xyz p))))
  Line(9)
  (EndAction) ]
```

If your tool allows attribute grammar descriptions, then you may be able to translate your attribute grammar directly.

Run your program with all the preceding programs. (You need no longer print out tokens and parse information.)

PSOOL Compiler Project Part 5
Symbol Table Creation

Average Time: 25–30 hours
Option 1 (Harder)

1. Add a symbol table to your program. Define its structure and a compiler switch to allow the printing of the symbol table after compilation.

2. Enhance your program to scan and parse programs described by the grammar of the previous assignment with the addition of declarations and array features as described by the following BNF.

3. Write your routines which access the symbol table as *abstract functions* and *procedures*. The calling procedures,

   ```
   enter (SymbolTable, Name)
   ```

   needn't know what the symbol table looks like.

5. Print by name *in alphabetical order*. If your data structure has a separate table for each class, you may print the information by class.

6. Use the word *Type* or *Class* for the symbol table attribute Class. Do not confuse this use of the word *Class* with the PSOOL language construct *Class*.

7. Symbol table attributes should include, at a minimum (more is better), the following headings:

Name	Type	Scope	Definition Line No.	Reference Line Nos.	Other
...					
Address Introduced	Class Variable	BankAccount	#		
Address	Class Variable	NOWAccount	#	#,#,#,#	
					Inherited from CheckingAccount
...					
HighInterestRate	Shared Variable	SavingsAccount	#	#, #, #	
					Inherited from BankAccount
...					
SavingsAccount	Class Name	BankAccount	#	#,#	

NEW BNF (Merge with old BNF)

```
Program → {ClassDescription}+  {Action}+
ClassDescription      →
   Class          ClassName ;
```

```
SuperClass
          SuperClassNames ;
                | None ;
InstanceVariables
    {Inherit    InheritClassNames ;
     From ClassName}⁺
                | None ;
    Introduce  IntroClassNames ;
                | None ;
SharedVariables
    {Inherit    SharedVarNames}
     From ClassName}⁺
                | None
    Introduce  SharedVarNames
                | None
  Methods       Methods|None
  EndClass      ClassName
Methods                    →
  Inherit    {InheritMethodNames
      From ClassName}⁺
             | None
  Introduce  IntroMethodNames
             | None
  Specialize{SpecializeMethodName
      With MethodName (Before
                     | After)}⁺
             | None
  Definitions     Definitions
             | None
Definitions          →
    {Method  MethodName
           (ParameterNames)
         LocalNames
              LocalNames
            | None
         BeginMethod
            SequenceOfStatements
     EndMethod  MethodName}⁺
```

Run your program on the following class descriptions (you may need to add a "dummy" action to the end of each or temporarily change the grammar to Program → {ClassDeclaration}⁺):

(a)

```
Class    Utilities ;
    SuperClass        None ;
    InstanceVariables
        Inherit       None ;
```

```
                Introduce      None ;
          SharedVariables
                Inherit        None ;
                Introduce      None ;
          Methods
                Inherit        None ;
                Introduce
                     Input,
                     PutPrompt ;
                Specialize     None ;
          Definitions
                Method Input (Info) ;
                  LocalNames  None ;
                  BeginMethod {Input}
                        Read(Info) ;
                EndMethod Input ;
                Method PutPrompt (Info) ;
                  LocalNames None ;
                  BeginMethod {PutPrompt}
                     Write (Info) ;
                EndMethod PutPrompt ;
       EndClass  Utilities ;
```

(b)

```
    Class    BankAccount ;
        SuperClass      None ;
        InstanceVariables
            Inherit    None ;
            Introduce
                Owner,
                Address,
                PhoneNumber,
                AccountNumber,
                Balance ;
        SharedVariables
            Inherit    None ;
            Introduce
                HighInterestRate := 0.07;
                LowInterestRate  := 0.045;
                NextAccountNumber:= 0;
        Methods
            Inherit    None ;
            Introduce
                GetInterestRate,
                DepositFunds,
                SetOwner,
```

```
                    SetAddress,
                    SetPhoneNumber,
                    GenerateAccountNumber ;
              Specialize    None ;
           Definitions
              Method GetInterestRate ;
                LocalNames None ;
                BeginMethod {GetInterestRate}
                If (Balance > 10000) Then
                Return (HighInterestRate) ;
                Else
                  Return (LowInterestRate) ;
                EndIf;
              EndMethod GetInterestRate ;
              Method DepositFunds ;
                    (AmountDeposited)
                LocalNames None ;
                BeginMethod {Deposit Funds}
                  Balance := Balance + AmountDeposited;
              EndMethod Deposit Funds ;
              Method SetOwner (Name) ;
                LocalNames None ;
                BeginMethod {SetOwner}
                  Owner := Name ;
              EndMethod SetOwner ;
              Method SetAddress(Name) ;
                LocalNames None ;
                BeginMethod {SetAddress}
                  Address := Name ;
              EndMethod SetAddress ;
              Method SetPhoneNumber (Number) ;
                LocalNames None ;
                BeginMethod {SetPhoneNumber}
                  PhoneNumber := Number ;
              EndMethod SetPhoneNumber ;
              Method GenerateAccountNumber ;
                LocalNames None ;
                BeginMethod
                  {GenerateAccountNumber}
                  NextAccountNumber := NextAccountNumber + 1 ;
                  AccountNumber := NextAccountNumber;
              EndMethod GenerateAccountNumber ;
         EndClass   BankAccount ;
```

(c)

```
Class SavingsAccount ;
    SuperClass
        BankAccount ;
    InstanceVariables
        Inherit
            Owner,
            Address,
            PhoneNumber,
            AccountNumber,
            Balance
        From BankAccount ;
        Introduce   None ;
    SharedVariables
        Inherit
            HighInterestRate := 0.07;
            LowInterestRate := 0.045;
            NextAccountNumber := 0;
        Introduce   None ;
    Methods
        Inherit
            GetInterestRate,
            DepositFunds,
            SetOwner,
            SetAddress,
            SetPhoneNumber,
            GenerateAccountNumber,
        From BankAccount ;
        Inherit
            Input,
            PutPrompt
        From Utilities ;
        Introduce   WithDrawFunds,
            AddInterestToBalance ;
        Specialize          None ;
     Definitions
        Method WithDrawFunds
            (AmountRequested) ;
            LocalNames IO ;
            BeginMethod {WithDrawFunds}
            If (AmountRequested >
                    Balance) Then
        New(Utilities);
            IO : PutPrompt ("Amount requested
                            higher than balance");
```

```
              Else Balance := Balance - Amount-
                                     Requested ;
              EndIf;
          EndMethod  WithdrawFunds ;
          Method AddInterestToBalance ;
           LocalNames InterestRate ;
           BeginMethod {AddInterestToBalance}
            InterestRate := self : GetInterestRate ;
            Balance := Balance +  Balance * Interest-
                                          Rate ;
           EndMethod  AddInterestToBalance ;
   EndClass    SavingsAccount ;
```

(d)

```
   Class   CheckingAccount ;
      SuperClass          BankAccount ;
      InstanceVariables
         Inherit
            Owner,
            Address,
            PhoneNumber,
            AccountNumber,
            Balance
         From BankAccount ;
       Introduce
            JointAccount,
            SecondAccountHolder ;
      SharedVariables
         Inherit
            HighInterestRate := 0.07;
            LowInterestRate  := 0.045;
            NextAccountNumber := 0 :
         From BankAccount
         Introduce
            BounceFee :=  12.50;
       Methods
         Inherit
            DepositFunds,
           {GetInterestRate removed}
            SetOwner,
            SetAddress,
            SetPhoneNumber,
            GenerateAccountNumber
         From BankAccount
         Introduce
            ClearCheck
```

```
        Specialize            None
          Definitions
          Method
          ClearCheck(CheckAmount)
          LocalNames None
             BeginMethod {ClearCheck}
             If (CheckAmount >
                   Balance) Then
             New(Utilities);
             IO : PutPrompt ("Amount requested higher
                            than balance");"
             Balance := Balance - BounceFee
             Else Balance := Balance - CheckAmount;
             EndIf
             EndMethod  ClearCheck
    EndClass  CheckingAccount
```

(e)

```
    Class    NOWAccount
        SuperClass
             SavingsAccount,
             CheckingAccount
        InstanceVariables
          Inherit
               Owner,
               Address,
               PhoneNumber,
               Balance,
               AccountNumber
               JointAccount,
               SecondAccountHolder
          From CheckingAccount
          Introduce   None
        SharedVariables
          Inherit
             HighInterestRate := 0.07;
             LowInterestRate  := 0.045;
             NextAccountNumber := 0;
          Introduce  None
        Methods
          Inherit
               GetInterestRate,
               DepositFunds,
               SetOwner,
               SetAddress,
               SetPhoneNumber,
```

```
              GenerateAccountNumber,
              WithDrawFunds,
              AddInterestToBalance
       From  Savings Account
       Inherit
              ClearCheck
       From     CheckingAccount
       Introduce     None
       Specialize
              GetInterestRate
       With CheckForMinimumBalance
       Before
     Definitions
       Method
         CheckForMinimumBalance
         LocalNames None
         BeginMethod
           {CheckForMinimumBalance}
            If (Balance < 1000) Then
               Return (0)
            EndIf
          EndMethod  CheckForMinimumBalance
     EndClass    NOWAccount
```

(f) A program of your choice

Arrays (see Appendix B, Part V) may also be added at this time.

Option 2 (Easier) Continue with the grammar of previous parts of the project.

$$\text{Program} \rightarrow \{\text{Action}\}^{+}$$

but implement more standard types than just integers (reals, characters, strings, and booleans, for example). This will require additions to the lexical analyzer and a change to the production for literals:

$$\text{Literal} \rightarrow \text{Integer} \,|\, \text{your additional types}$$

Implement your symbol table as described in Option 1. Create programs which test these types.

PSOOL Compiler Project Part 6
Code Lowering ***Optional***

This assignment is completely optional. It also could be done at the same time as Part 5.

Now that information about names is stored in the symbol table, information about them can be removed from the abstract syntax trees. This will make it easier to scan the tree during code generation.

Thus, the first example program might produce the following output:

```
[
  Line(4)
  (:=
     (a, b3))
  (:=
   Line(5-6)
   (xyz, +
           (a +
              (b -
                 (c /
                    (p q))))))
  Line(7)
  (:=
        (a *
           (xyz +
               (p  q))))
  Line(8)
  (:=
     (p -
        (a  -
           (xyz  p))))
  Line(9)
  (EndAction)]
```

It will also ease the code generation if high-level statements such as WHILE loops are "lowered to their "IF statement" form. For example,

```
(WHILE
    (=
       (I  J)
    (:=
        (I  +
            (I 2)))))
```

can be changed to (something like):

```
(Label L1)
(IF
   (≠
      ((I J)  (GO L2)
      (:=
          .(I  +
              (I 2))))
(GO L1)
(Label L2)
```

7

Optimization: Introduction and Control Flow Analysis

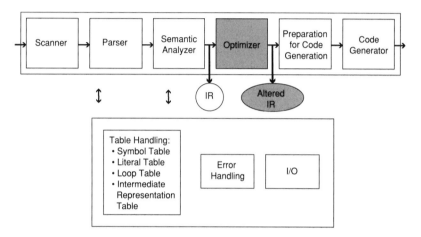

7.0 Introduction

The optimization phase makes changes to the intermediate representation so that the code generator will put out better but equivalent code.

The term *optimization* is a misnomer. The problem of changing code in all cases to the best it can be is an *undecidable* problem; it cannot be solved by an algorithm on a computer.

We can, however, *improve* code in most cases.

There are machine dependent optimizations such as good allocation of registers and machine independent optimizations such as computing constants; constant computation at compile-time rather than generating code to compute them saves execution time.

Optimization can consume a lot of compile-time, so we want the most payoff for the least effort. In particular, the compiler needs to guess where the most frequently executed parts of the program are.

7.1 Comparison of Algorithms

Optimization can't speed up a really slow algorithm by large factors. Figure 1 shows, within multiplication by a constant, the amount of data which can be processed relative to a base value. If 1000 "widgets" can be processed in linear time, then only 140 can be processed using an algorithm which is O(nlogn), etc.

Time Complexity	Maximum Problem Size		
	1 Second	1 Minute	1 Hour
n	1000	6×10^4	3.6×10^6
nlogn	140	4893	2×10^5
n^2	31	244	1897
n^3	10	39	150
2^n	9	15	21

Figure 1

Suppose we are able to optimize a program to produce a speed-up of a factor of 10 (an ambitious improvement).

If we let S = problem size, then after a speed-up by a factor of 10:

Complexity	**Problem Size**
Linear (n)	10S
nlogn	10S (for large S)
n^2	3.16S
n^3	2.15S
2^n	S + 3.3

We can conclude from this that bad algorithms are not helped much by optimization.

However, clever optimizations of clever code may not improve things either. Knuth (1971) presented an amusing discussion in which he refered to an algorithm which he had developed many years ago which translated a complicated expression to fewer instructions than some other people's algorithm. Years later, he realized that programmers rarely used such complicated expressions, and it isn't worth the compiler's time to optimize them.

7.2   What to Optimize

We want to optimize things that happen frequently. There are two kinds of *frequently*: (1) how frequently a piece of code is ever written and (2) how frequently a piece of code is executed within a program.

For (1), Knuth (1971) shows empirically that simple assignment statements with one operation and one to three variables are the most often used statements:

```
A := B
A := A Op 1
A := A Op k
A := B Op k
A := B Op C
```

Here, A, B, and, C are variables and k is a constant. Follow-up studies have continued to confirm this. It does little good to optimize for things programmers rarely write.

For (2), code in loops tends to be executed the most; thus optimizations concentrate on loops.

7.3 Issues in Optimization

The most important optimization principle is *correctness*. The meaning of a program can't be changed:

Principle 1. If you can't do it safely, don't do it.

The task is to find frequently occurring code sequences, perform improvements to them, and forget the rest.

Principle 2. Don't expect the programmer to optimize high-level language features.

Sometimes the questions are asked: *Why optimize? Can't programmers just be taught to write good code?* The answer is (rarely) *yes*. For large programs which execute for many hours or days, programmers do rewrite them to make them as efficient as possible. The more common answer, however, is *no*. Programmers should be able to use the features of a language to implement an algorithm without worrying about its efficiency. They should be optimizing for readability and maintainability. Example 1 shows a common case

EXAMPLE 1   Two-dimensional arrays

```
LOOP
  A[I,J] := . . .
  . . .
  . . .
   := A[I,J]
  . . .
ENDLOOP
```

The translated code for Example 1 quite likely has "things" which can be optimized. The programmer could conceivably do it—by using one-dimensional arrays, etc. Realistically, then, the programmer might as well not be using a high-level language.

An optimizing compiler is *expected* to optimize the high-level features.

Optimizations optimize most frequently for *time*. This is represented, syntactically (that is, it can be seen by looking at the code), by minimization of the number of operations and minimization of the number of memory accesses. Operations can be computed faster if their operands are in registers. Constants can be computed at compile-time.

Optimizations optimize next most frequently for *space*. Minimizing memory accesses may produce a smaller amount of code as well as code that executes faster since most machine code requires more bytes to reference memory.

There are also space-time tradeoffs. For example, replacing two instances of the same code by a subroutine may save code space, but takes more time because of the overhead of jumping to the subroutine, passing arguments and returning from the subroutine.

An optimization should speed up a program by a measurable amount. Also, we don't optimize in heavy debugging environments (student environments are heavy debugging environments). It takes too much compiler time for environments where a program is compiled many times (until it is correct) and run once or twice.

On the other hand, as we shall see, certain so-called peephole optimizations are so easy that they should be done by all compilers.

7.4   Optimization Phases

Optimization can be performed on the tree. This is called high-level optimization. Even with today's programming standards—no transfer into the middle of loops, etc.—principle 1 makes these high-level optimizations unsafe. We will see why when we look at a formal definition of a loop. More aggressive, as well as correct, optimizations are made on a graphical intermediate representation of a program.

The phase which represents the pertinent, possible flow of control is often called *control flow analysis*. If this representation is graphical, then a *flow graph* depicts *all* possible execution paths. Control flow analysis simplifies the data flow analysis. Data flow analysis is the process of collecting information about the *modification*, *preservation*, and *use* of program "quantities"—usually *variables* and *expressions*.

Once control flow analysis and data flow analysis have been done, the next phase, the improvement phase, improves the program code so that it runs faster or uses less space. This phase is sometimes termed *optimization*. Thus, the term optimization is used for this final code improvement, as well as for the entire process which includes control flow analysis and data flow analysis.

Optimization algorithms attempt to remove useless code, eliminate redundant expressions, move invariant computations out of loops, etc.

The next section describes control flow analysis. We begin by creating the control flow graph.

7.5   Control Flow Analysis

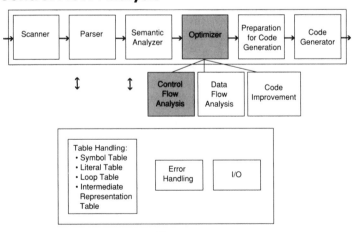

Figure 2

Control flow analysis proceeds in two steps: (1) determine the basic blocks— sequences of straight-line code and (2) build a flow graph by taking branches into account.

7.5.1   Basic Blocks

A *basic block* is a sequence of intermediate representation constructs (quadruples, abstract syntax trees, whatever) which allow no flow of control *in* or *out* of the block except at the top or bottom. Figure 3 shows the structure of a basic block.

Figure 3

We will use the term *statement* for the intermediate representation and show it in quadruple form because quadruples are easier to read than IR in tree form.

Leaders

A basic block consists of a *leader* and all code before the next leader. We define a *leader* to be (1) the first statement in the program (or procedure), (2) the target of a branch, identified most easily because it has a label, and (3) the statement after a "diverging flow": the statement after a conditional or unconditional branch. Figure 4 shows this pictorially:

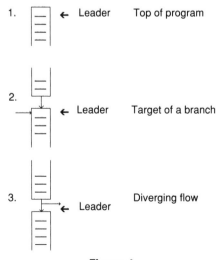

Figure 4

Basic blocks can be built during parsing if it is assumed that all labels are referenced or after parsing without that assumption. Example 2 shows the outline of a FOR-Loop and its basic blocks.

Since a basic block consists of straight-line code, it computes a set of expressions. Many optimizations are really transformations applied to basic blocks and to sequences of basic blocks.

EXAMPLE 2   Basic blocks for a FOR-Loop

```
FOR I := 1 TO N DO
     S₁;
ENDFOR
S₂
```

The basic blocks and their leaders are:

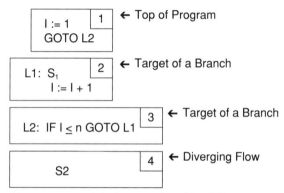

Although this program might be translated in different ways, the discussion here is still valid.

Once we have computed basic blocks, we can create the control flow graph.

7.5.2   Building a Flow Graph

A flow graph shows all possible execution paths. We will use this information to perform optimizations.

Formally, a *flow graph* is a directed graph G, with N nodes and E edges. (Remember that a *directed graph* is a connected set of *nodes* where every node is reachable from the initial node.) Example 3 shows the control flow graph for Example 2. The rules for building such a graph follow.

EXAMPLE 3   Building the control flow graph

```
FOR I := 1 TO n DO
     S₁
ENDFOR
S₂
```

                              ↓

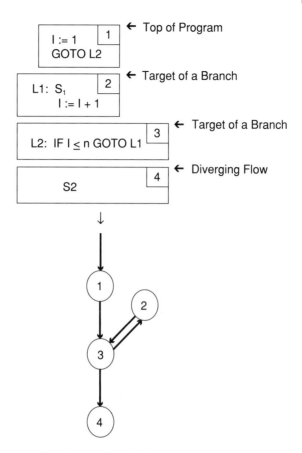

In Example 3, we see that the set of *nodes* is the set of basic blocks and the set of edges is determined by looking at places where the nodes branch.

More formally, we create nodes and arcs as shown in Figure 5. Successors and predecessors are defined as in Figure 5.

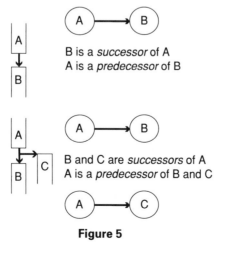

Figure 5

These are *all* the edges in a flow graph. (Convince yourself of this.)

7.5.3 Techniques for Building Flow Graphs

Building a control flow graph involves finding predecessors and successors.

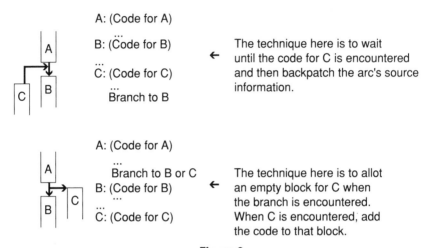

Figure 6

Consider the first situation of Figure 6 where basic block A has been built and a leader is identified for the beginning of basic block B. We cannot build the tail of the arrow to basic block B until we find the diverging flow that leads here. *Backpatching:* returning and filling in the tail information, will define the source of this arc.

The second picture represents the opposite situation. In the second picture in Figure 6, we know we have an arc, but haven't found the leader to which the arc should point; the tail of the arc is known, but its head is not. Here, we can allocate a data structure for a basic block and then backpatch when it is found.

7.5.4 Data Structures for Building Control Flow Graphs

Basic blocks may be created and destroyed as the program is modified in the optimization process. Thus, space must be made available for growing collections of blocks. Storage reclamation is essential to handle optimization of large programs.

Since the structure of the flow graph varies with time, the data structure for blocks might keep pointers to lists of successors.

Since statements within the block change with time, it is reasonable to keep the intermediate representation as a linked list and reclaim storage of unused statements. Another possibility is to allocate dynamically on a heap and then garbage collect (see a data structures text if the terms *heap* and *garbage collection* are not familiar) when the heap runs out. See Chapter 11 for a discussion of garbage collection.

7.5.5 DAGs

The previous sections looked at the control flow graph nodes of basic blocks. DAGs, on the other hands, create a useful structure for the intermediate representation *within* the basic blocks.

A directed graph with no cycles, called a *DAG* (Directed Acyclic Graph), is used to represent a basic block. Thus, the nodes of a flow graph are themselves graphs! We can create a DAG *instead of* an abstract syntax tree by modifying the operations for constructing the nodes. If the node already exists, the operation returns a pointer to the existing node. Example 4 shows this for the two-line assignment statement example.

EXAMPLE 4   A DAG for two assignment statements

```
X1 := a + bb * 12 ;
X2 := a/2 + bb * 12 ;
```

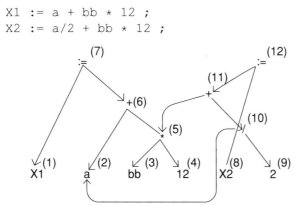

In Example 4, there are two references to *a* and two references to the quantity *bb * 12.*

7.5.6   Data Structure for a DAG

As Example 4 shows, each node may have more than one pointer to it. We can represent a DAG internally by a process known as *value-numbering*. Each node is numbered and this number is entered whenever this node is reused. This is shown in Example 5.

EXAMPLE 5   Value-numbering

Node	Left Child	Right Child
1. X1		
2. a		
3. bb		
4. 12		
5. *	(3)	(4)
6. +	(2)	(5)
7. :=	(1)	(6)
8. X2		
9. 2		
10. /	(2)	(9)
11. +	(10)	(5)
12. :=	(8)	(11)

7.5.7 Benefits of DAGs

When a DAG is created, common subexpressions are detected. Also, creating a DAG makes it easy to see variables and expressions which are used or defined within a block.

DAGs also produce good code at code generation time. In Chapter 10, we will see a code generation algorithm which produces good (but not optimal!) code from a DAG.

Example 6 shows a bubble sort procedure and a set of quadruples to which it might be translated. *Quadruples* are an intermediate representation consisting of a single operation, up to two operands and a result. They are easier for humans to read than an abstract syntax tree.

EXAMPLE 6   IR for a bubble sort procedure

```
FOR I := 1 TO n - 1 DO
    FOR J := 1 TO I DO
        IF A[J] > A[J + 1] THEN
            BEGIN
                Temp := A[J]
                A[J] := A[ J + 1 ]
                A[J + 1] := Temp
            END
                ↓
            I := 1
            GOTO ITest
ILoop:  J := 1
            GOTO JTest
JLoop:  T1 := 4 * J
            T2 := A[T1]      ; A[J]
            T3 := J + 1
            T4 := 4 * T3
            T5 := A[T4]      ; A[J + 1]
            IF T2 ≤ T5 GOTO JPlus
            T6 := 4 * J
            Temp := A[T6]  ; Temp := A[J]
            T7 := J + 1
            T8 := 4 * T7
            T9 := A[T8]      ; A[J + 1]
            T10 := 4 * J
            A[T10] := T9     ; A[J] := A[J + 1]
            T11 := J + 1
            T12 := 4 * T11
            A[T12] := Temp ; A[J + 1] := Temp
JPlus:  J := J + 1
JTest:  IF J ≤ I GOTO JLoop
IPlus:  I := I + 1
ITest:  IF I ≤ n - 1 GOTO ILoop
```

The intermediate code shown in Example 6 is rather high-level. For machines which have no indexing modes, the references to A[...] will have to be computed by the compiler. Also, the IF statements really involve several quadruples (see Chapter 6). The multiplication by "4" could, alternatively, be done at code generation time. We do it here because it will give us more opportunities for optimization of our example.

Using "( )" to mean "contents of" and "addr" to mean "address of", the low-level quadruples for "Temp := List[i]" might be:

```
T1  := addr(List)
T2  := T1 + I
Temp := (T2)
```

Similarly, if the array reference is on the left-hand side of an assignment statement as in "List[I] := Temp", low-level quadruples would be:

```
T1  := addr(List)
T2  := T1 + I
(T2) := Temp
```

Even if a machine has an indexing addressing mode, translating array references into their low-level format may allow optimizations (for example, if the subscript reference were a common subexpression).

Nevertheless, there will be numerous opportunities to improve the code sequence in Example 6.

Example 7 shows the basic blocks and the control flow graph for the procedure in Example 6.

EXAMPLE 7   Control flow graph for a bubble sort

```
           I := 1                << Block 1
           GOTO ITest
ILoop:     J := 1                << Block 2
           GOTO JTest
JLoop:     T1 := 4 * J           << Block 3
           T2 := A[T1]    ; A[J]
           T3 := J + 1
           T4 := 4 * T3
           T5 := A[T4]    ; A[J + 1]
           IF T2 ≤ T5 GOTO JPlus
           T6 := 4 * J           << Block 4
           Temp := A[T6] ; Temp := A[J]
           T7 := J + 1
           T8 := 4 * T7
           T9 := A[T8]    ; A[J + 1]
           T10 := 4 * J
           A[T10] := T9   ; A[J] := A[J + 1]
           T11 := J + 1
```

```
             T12 := 4 * T11
             A[T12] := Temp ; A[J + 1] := Temp
JPlus:       J := J + 1              << Block 5
JTest:       IF J ≤ I GOTO JLoop     << Block 6
IPlus:       I := I + 1              << Block 7
ITest:       IF I ≤ n - 1 GOTO ILoop << Block 8
```

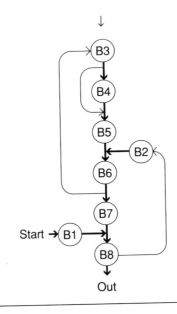

Example 8 shows a DAG for block 3 of Example 7.

EXAMPLE 8   DAG for block 3

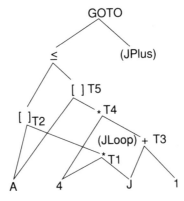

The program of Example 7 contains cycles which may be loops. Determining loops is a major activity of control flow analysis. Creating basic blocks and a control flow graph are two steps toward this process. In the next section, we will formalize the process of determining a loop in a control flow graph.

7.6 Loops

Programs spend the bulk of their time in loops. Thus, the payoff in loop optimization is potentially high.

There are two main types of loop optimizations: (1) movement of loop-invariant computations outside of the loop and (2) elimination of excess induction variables, the variables which are a linear function of the loop index. Other optimizations often performed within loops are reductions in strength of certain multiplications to additions.

Example 9 shows invariant code movement. The details of how this optimization is found and implemented are given in the next two chapters. In this chapter we focus on the importance of being able to identify a loop.

EXAMPLE 9   Invariant code motion

```
FOR index := 1 TO 10000 DO        t := y * z
BEGIN                             FOR index:= 1 TO 10000 DO
   x := y * z ;                   BEGIN
   j := index * 3 ;        →         x := t
END                                  j := index * 3
 .                                END
 .                                 .
                                   .
                                   .
```

In Example 9, $y * z$ is computed each time around the loop. If none of y, z, or x changes value in the loop (and this must be checked!), then it is more efficient to compute this product, t, once and to use t every place the computation appears in the loop (x itself may be able to be be eliminated).

Example 9 can also be optimized for strength reduction (turn the multiplication into an addition) and for elimination of induction variables (*index* and *j* are tracking one another). We will save these examples for Chapter 9.

7.6.1   Defining a Loop

In order to have a method for finding loops suitable for optimization (not all are), we need to define what a loop is.

Intuitively, cycles in flow graphs are loops, but to perform optimizations we need a second property:

A loop must have a single entry point

7.6.2   Headers

A node n is the *header* of a set of nodes S if every path from the start node to a node in S first goes through n.

A cycle must have a header to be considered a loop. Optimizations such as code motion cannot be done safely if there is more than one entry to the loop. Also, the header concept makes the algorithms for loop-invariant code motion, etc. conceptually simpler.

Example 10 shows a flow graph with two cycles, one of which *is* a loop and one of which *is not* a loop.

EXAMPLE 10   A loop and not a loop

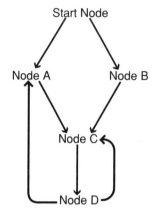

In Example 10, {*Node C, Node D*} is a loop with header *Node C*. The cycle {*Node A, Node C, Node D*} is not a loop because we can enter the cycle at both *Node A* and *Node C*.

Finding Loops

Although the preceding definition is helpful for us humans to find a loop, we will need some more definitions in order to write an algorithm to find a loop.

An efficient algorithm for finding a loop involves finding *dominators, depth-first search,* and *depth-first* ordering.

7.6.3   Dominators

A node *d dominates* a node *n*, written *d DOM n*, if every path from the start node to *n* goes through *d*. This means that a node dominates itself. Example 11 shows dominators for the graph of Example 10.

EXAMPLE 11   Dominators

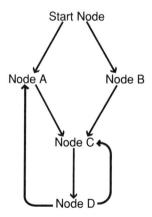

> Here, the *Start* node dominates all nodes; *Node A* and *Node B* do not dominate anything except themselves, *Node C* dominates *Node D* and itself, and *Node D* does not dominate anything except itself.

Note that for a node to dominate a node *n*, it must be *n* or dominate every predecessor of *n*. We use this fact to create an algorithm to find the dominators in a control flow graph. We use the notation *Dom(n)* for the set of dominators of a node *n*.

Algorithm
Finding Dominators

```
DOM(Start) := {Start}
FOR node ≠ Start DO
    DOM(node) = {All nodes}
ENDFOR
WHILE changes to any DOM(node) occur DO
        FOR each node ≠ start DO
            DOM(node) := {node} ∪ ( ∩ Dom(p) )
                                  p ε Pred(node)
        ENDFOR
ENDWHILE
```

This algorithm for computing dominators does not indicate in what order to visit the node, just that all nodes are visited. In a later section, we will discuss an order for which this algorithm converges rapidly. Example 12 shows dominators being calculated for the graph of Example 11.

EXAMPLE 12   Calculation of dominators for example graph

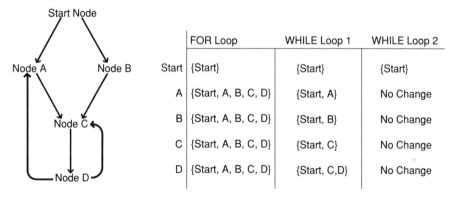

		FOR Loop	WHILE Loop 1	WHILE Loop 2
	Start	{Start}	{Start}	{Start}
	A	{Start, A, B, C, D}	{Start, A}	No Change
	B	{Start, A, B, C, D}	{Start, B}	No Change
	C	{Start, A, B, C, D}	{Start, C}	No Change
	D	{Start, A, B, C, D}	{Start, C,D}	No Change

In Example 12, the correct value of the dominators is found in the first pass through the WHILE loop. One more pass is needed to discover that there are no changes.

7.6.4 Natural Loops

We use dominators to find loops. Since loops contain a cycle, and a header dominates all the nodes in a loop,

> there must be at least one arc entering the header from a node in the
> loop

For this reason, we search for an arc whose head dominates its tail. This is called
a *back edge*. Loops must have a back edge.

The *natural loop* of the back edge is defined to be the *smallest set of nodes* that
includes the back edge and has no predecessors outside the set except for the predecessor of the header. Natural loops are the loops for which we find optimizations.

Algorithm
Finding the nodes in a natural loop

```
FOR every node n, find all m such that n DOM m
FOR every back edge t → h, i.e., for every arc such that
    h DOM t, construct the natural loop:
        Delete h and find all nodes which can lead to t
These nodes plus h form the natural loop of t → h
```

EXAMPLE 13   Finding a natural loop

Start DOM Start
Start DOM A
Start DOM B
Start DOM C
Start DOM D

A DOM A
B DOM B
C DOM C
C DOM D
D DOM D

Back edge D → C
D leads to D

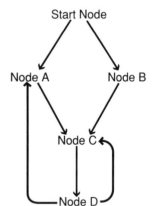

Natural loop is {C, D}

The only back edge in Example 13 is Node D → Node C. It is a back
edge since Node C DOM Node D, that is, the head, Node C, dominates
the tail, Node D. When Node C is deleted, no other node leads to Node D.
Thus {Node C, Node D} is a natural loop.

Step 1 in the algorithm for finding a natural loop does not say *how* to
find dominators, nor does the algorithm for finding dominators say in
which order to visit the nodes. Visiting the nodes in a depth-first order
tends to find the dominators and expose back edges faster.

7.6.5 Depth-First Order and Depth-First Spanning Trees

Intuitively, we begin at the start node and attempt to get as far away as possible. As we proceed, we can make a (yet another!) tree from the arcs of the flow graph. This is called a *depth-first spanning tree, DFST.*

A *depth-first order* is defined to be the reverse of the order in which we last visit the nodes of the control graph when we create the DFST. The following algorithm creates a depth-first spanning tree.

Algorithm
DFST
```
T := empty
n := Start node
REPEAT
    IF n has an unmarked successor s THEN
    BEGIN
        Add n → s to T
        Mark s
        n := s
    END
    ELSE
        n := parent of n in T
UNTIL n = start node and n has no unmarked successors
```

EXAMPLE 14   Finding a DFST

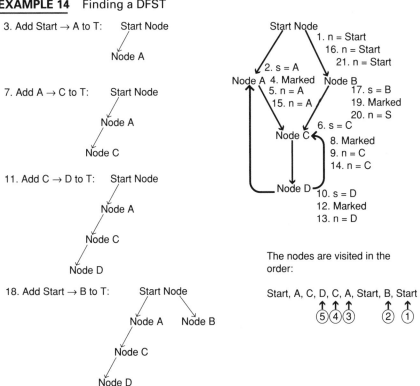

The nodes are visited in the order:

Start, A, C, D, C, A, Start, B, Start

The circled numbers in Example 14 point to the reverse of the order in which we last visit the nodes. A depth-first order here is *Start, Node B, Node A, Node C, Node D* (the reverse of the order in which we last visited the nodes while creating the DFST). It is not the only depth-first order nor is this the only depth-first spanning tree (see Exercise 6).

Exercise 4 asks the readers to compute dominators by visiting the nodes in a somewhat random order and then to compute dominators by visiting the nodes in a depth-first order. For some graphs, the algorithm terminates faster when the nodes are visited in a depth-first order than when they are visited in the order *Start, Node A, Node B, Node C, Node D*.

7.6.6   Finding Natural Loops Efficiently

We introduce one more definition—a *backwards edge*.

To find the loops of a program efficiently:

1. Compute a depth-first order (DFO). The *backwards edges* are those whose heads precede their tails in the DFO.

2. Compute dominators. The *back edges* are the *backwards edges* whose heads dominate their tails.

3. For each back edge, compute the *natural loop*.

These steps find the natural loops of a program in an efficient way.

7.7   Summary

This chapter has introduced optimization and a graphical representation of a program called a control flow graph. One of the main reasons a control flow graph is created is to be able to find a loop suitable for optimizations involving code motion. For structured programs which have a single entry to and exit from a loop, a loop can be identified from the nodes of an abstract syntax tree. Even newer languages such as Ada, however, allow a loop to be exited in more than one place. The Related Reading references papers which find control flow on higher-level constructs such as trees and a method of loop finding called interval analysis.

7.8   Related Reading

Aho, A. V. and J. D. Ullman. 1975. *Listings for Reducible Flow Graphs*, 7th ACM Symposium on Theory of Computing, 177–185.

Allen, F. E. 1970. Control Flow Analysis, *SIGPLAN Notices*, 5(7):1–19.

Cytron, R., A. Lowry, and K. Zadeck. 1986. *Code Motion of Control Structures in High-Level Languages*, Proceedings of the 13th POPL Conference, 70–85.

Garey, M. R. and D. S. Johnson. 1979. *Computers and Intractability—A Guide to the Theory of NP-Completeness*, San Francisco: W. H. Freeman.

Hecht, M S. 1977. *Flow Analysis of Computer Programs*, New York: Elsevier North-Holland.

Knuth, D. E. 1971. An Empirical Study of FORTRAN Programs, *Software Practice and Experience*, 1:105–133.

Muchnick, S. and N. Jones, Eds. 1979. *Program Flow Analysis: Theory and Applications*, Englewood, Cliffs, NJ: Prentice-Hall, 79–101.

Tarjan, R. E. 1974. Testing Flow Graph Reducibility, *Journal of Computer and System Sciences*, 9:355–365.

EXERCISES

1. For the following program, compute (a) a quadruple intermediate representation, (b) the basic blocks, (c) the control flow graph (d) back edges, and (e) natural loops.

```
PROGRAM Plus
   BEGIN {Plus}
   LOOP FOR I := 1 TO L DO
     BEGIN {I Loop}
     LOOP FOR J := 1 TO M DO
       BEGIN {J Loop}
         Z[I,J] := X[I,J] + Y[I,J]
       END {J Loop}
     END {ILoop}
   END {Plus}
```

2. For the program of Example 6, find (a) dominators, (b) back edges, and (c) natural loops.

3. (a) Create a DAG for

```
I := I + 10
J := I + 10
```

   (b) Represent the nodes using value-numbering.
   (c) What optimization is exposed by creating the DAG here?

4. For the following graph, compute dominators (a) by visiting the nodes in numerical order and (b) by visiting them in depth-first order.

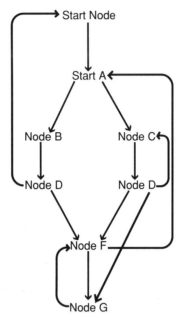

5. For the following program, find (a) quadruples, (b) basic blocks, (c) the control flow graph, (d) a depth-first order, (e) dominators, (f) back edges, (g) natural loops.

```
PROGRAM Mult
   BEGIN {Mult}
     LOOP FOR I := 1 TO L DO
     BEGIN {I Loop}
       LOOP FOR J := 1 TO N DO
       BEGIN {J Loop}
         Z[I,J] := 0
       LOOP FOR K := 1 TO M DO
         BEGIN {K Loop}
           Z[I,J] := X[I,K] * Y[K,J] + Z[I,J]
         END {KLoop}
       END {JLoop}
     END {ILoop}
   END {Mult}
```

6. For Example 14, find another depth-first order and another depth-first spanning tree.

Project

The next, and last, phase of the compiler project is the code generation phase. The projects from Chapter 6 will take awhile to complete.

8

Optimization: Data Flow Analysis

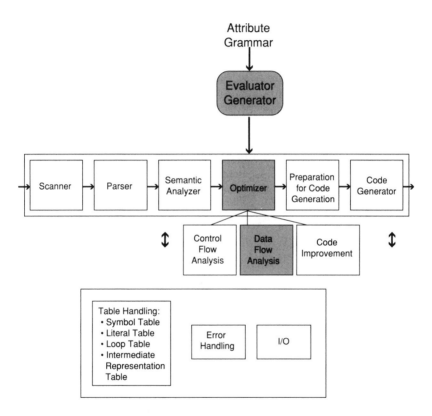

8.0   Introduction

Data flow analysis provides information regarding the *definition* and *use* of data items. It provides the following information (among others): (1) paths along which a reference to a data item is not preceded by a definition and (2) detection of redundant or useless code. As the diagram above shows, we approach data flow analysis in two ways. The first, a low-level approach, is from a compiler phase perspective, using the control flow graph intermediate representation developed in Chapter 7. The second, a high-level approach, is to evaluate attributes on the abstract syntax tree.

Example 1 shows some problems which may be exposed by data flow analysis.

EXAMPLE 1

> (1)
>   x := 3 (unused definition)
>   x := 2
> (2)
>   x := 3 (useless assignment)
>   (no ... := x)
> (3)
>   A := 3 (identical variables)
>   B := 3

In addition to those shown in Example 1, loop invariant variables may be detected, expressions which have already been computed may be detected, etc.

8.1   Data Flow Analysis Methods

We can gather relevant information for data flow analysis in a way similar to the way gossip is propagated: locally available information is initially posted and then propagated over the possible paths in the control graph.

Most data flow problems can be defined by equations. Iterative techniques are used to solve these equations. Example 2 shows a typical problem.

EXAMPLE 2   Typical data flow problem

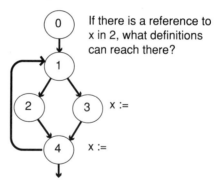

If there is a reference to x in 2, what definitions can reach there?

8.1.1   The Problem

Given a control flow structure, we want to discern which *definitions* of program quantities can affect which *uses* within the program.

Data flow problems fall into two classes. First are those which, given a point in the program, ask what can happen *before* control reaches that point—that is, what (past) *definitions* can affect computations at that point. We call these *forward flow* problems.

Second are those which, given a point in the program, ask what can happen *after* control leaves that point—that is, what (future) *uses* can be affected by computations at that point. We call these *backward flow* problems.

Forward flow problems include *reaching definitions* and *available expressions.* Backward flow problems include *live variable* analysis, *very busy expressions,* and *reached uses.*

We will examine these one by one.

8.2   Reaching Definitions

Reaching definitions determine for each basic block B and each program variable x what statements of the program could be the last statement defining x along some path from the start node to B.

A statement *defines x* if it assigns a value to x, for example, an assignment or read of x, or a procedure call passed x (not by value) or a procedure call that can access x.

Formally, we say that a definition, *def*

```
def: x :=
```

reaches a point p in the program if there is some path from the start node to p along which *def* occurs and, subsequent to *def,* there are no other definitions of x. Figure 1 shows this pictorially.

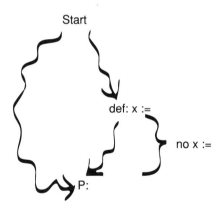

Figure 1

8.2.1   Data Flow Equations

For data flow analysis problems, we create and solve a collection of data flow equations. The *variables* are

```
In(B) and Out(B)
```

for a given block *B*.

There are two classes of equations:

1. A *transfer equation* to transfer data within the blocks
2. A *confluence rule* to transfer data when paths come together

8.2.2   Transfer Equation for Reaching Definitions

For all forward flow problems, the information which comes out of the block is a function of the information which goes into the block. We write this symbolically as:

```
Out(B) = f_B(In(B))
```

For *reaching definitions*, we define function f in terms of definitions which are *generated* and *killed* in the block B. We thus introduce two new variables: *Kill(B)* and *Gen(B)*.

Definition def_1 kills definition def_2 if def_1 and def_2 define the same variable:

```
Kill(B) = The set of definitions in the other blocks
          of the program that are killed by some
          definition in B.
```

Block B *generates* definition *def* if *def* is in B and is the last definition of *def*'s variable within B.

```
Gen(B) = set of definitions generated by B
```

The transfer equation is:

```
Out(B) = (In(B) - Kill(B)) ∪ Gen(B)
```

Confluence Rule for Reaching Definitions

A definition *def* reaches the beginning of a block B if and only if it reaches the end of one of block B's predecessors.

```
In(B) = ∪ Out(P)
      P ∈ Pred(B)
```

EXAMPLE 3   Reaching definitions

Start

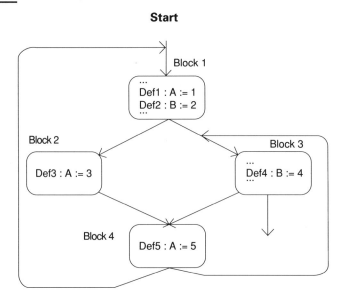

Using the preceding definitions for Gen and Kill, we have, for Example 3:

```
Gen(Block1) = {Def1,Def2}
                        Kill(Block1) = {Def3,Def4,Def5}
Gen(Block2) = {Def3} Kill(Block2) = {Def1,Def5}
Gen(Block3) = {Def4} Kill(Block3) = {Def2}
Gen(Block4) = {Def5} Kill(Block4) = {Def1,Def3}
```

Using the transfer equation, the Out's equations are:

1. Out(Block1) =
      (In(Block1) − {Def3,Def4,Def5}) ∪ {Def1,Def2}
2. Out(B2) = (In(B2) − {Def1,Def5}) ∪ {Def3}
3. Out(B3) = (In(B3) − {Def2}) ∪ {Def4}
4. Out(B4) = (In(B4) − {Def1,Def3}) ∪ {Def5}

Using the confluence rule, the In equations are:

5. In(B1) = Out(B4)
6. In(B2) = Out(B1)
7. In(B3) = Out(B1) ∪ Out(B4)
8. In(B4) = Out(B2) ∪ Out(B3)

Although we have eight equations in eight unknowns, techniques from algebra such as Gaussian Elimination cannot be applied since the values of the unknown must be taken from an algebraic field. (What would `{Def1,Def2}/2` or `1/{Def1}` even mean?)

But these equations do have a least solution, and this is the solution we want. We find it by iteration.

8.2.3 The Iterative Method for Solving Data Flow Equations

We will develop an iterative algorithm for reaching definitions. The reader need not despair that there will be a new algorithm for every data flow problem, however. Only minor changes need to be made to the equation to solve the other problems.

We start by assuming that what comes out of a block consists of the definitions generated in them.

We then repeatedly visit the nodes, applying the *confluence* rules to get new *In*'s and the *transfer* rules to get new *Out*'s. By *pred(B)*, we mean the immediate predecessors.

Algorithm
Reaching Definitions
```
FOR each block B, DO
  In(B) = φ
  Out(B) = Gen(B)
ENDFOR
  WHILE there are changes DO
    FOR each block B DO
```

```
In(B)  =  ∪ Out(P)
          P ∈ Pred(B)

Out(B)  =  (In(B) − Kill(B)) ∪ Gen(B)
      ENDFOR
ENDWHILE
```

EXAMPLE 4   Reaching Definitions for Example 3

	Block 1	Block 2	Block 3	Block 4
FOR Loop	In = φ Out = {Def1,Def2}	In = φ Out = {Def3}	In = φ Out = {Def4}	In = φ Out = Def5
WHILE Loop Iteration 1	In = {Def5} Out = {Def1,Def2}	In = {Def1,Def2} Out = {Def2,Def3}	In = {Def1,Def2,Def5} Out = {Def1,Def4,Def5}	In = {Def1—Def5} Out = {Def2,Def4,Def5}
WHILE Loop Iteration 2	In = {Def2,Def4,Def5} Out = {Def1,Def2}	In = {Def1,Def2} Out = {Def2,Def3}	In = {Def1,Def2,Def4,Def5} Out = {Def1,Def4,Def5}	In = {Def1—Def5} Out = {Def2,Def4,Def5}
WHILE Loop Iteration 3	In = {Def2,Def4,Def5} Out = {Def1,Def2}	In = {Def1,Def2} Out = {Def2,Def3}	In = {Def1,Def2,Def4,Def5} Out = {Def1,Def4,Def5}	In = {Def1—Def5} Out = {Def2,Def4,Def5}

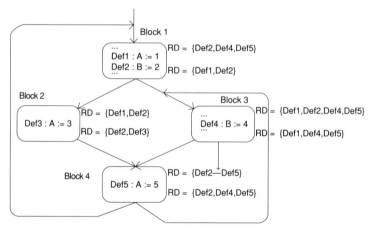

The values in the first set of Example 4 are the values computed using the FOR Loop and using the definitions of Gen above. In the third iteration of the WHILE Loop, the values are the same as for the second iteration; thus there are no changes and the final solution is found. The control flow graph is labeled with the final result.

8.2.4   Data Structures for Reaching Definitions

Most of the space for these is devoted to storing the *In(B)* and *Out(B)* sets. These sets are a subset of all variable definitions.

We could represent a definition by a pointer to its text, but the *In, Out* sets may be large.

A better way is to number the definitions and create a table whose *ith* entry points to the *ith* definition. The *In* and *Out* sets can then be bit vectors such that the *ith* position is set if the ith definition is in the set.

Other space improvements include limiting the variables to be considered and then we can limit the length of the bit vectors.

For the bit vector operations, union can be implemented by a Boolean *or,* intersection by *and,* and set difference by *and not.*

8.2.5   Application of Reaching Definitions

Not all uses of data flow analysis involve code optimization. We can use reaching definitions to detect possible uses of variables before they have been defined. Detecting (at compile time) statements that use a variable before its definition is a useful debugging aid.

To adapt reaching definitions to solve this:

(i) Introduce a new dummy block D that contains a definition of each variable used in the program.
(ii) Place D before the Start node.
(iii) Compute reaching definitions.
(iv) If any definition in D reaches B where the variable is used, then we have a *use* before a *definition.*

In some languages, we should print a warning. In other languages, however, a default initial value may be assumed, and although a warning message could be issued, it would be incorrect not to generate the code for the program.

8.3   Available Expressions

Available expressions make use of an expression *used* in one block which was *computed* in another block. Thus, at code generation time, code to recompute the expression need not be emitted. Example 5 shows an expression *BB * 12* which is computed on all paths leading to *X3.*

EXAMPLE 5   An available expression

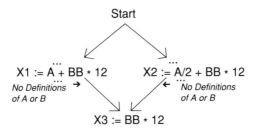

In Example 5, the expression *BB * 12* is available for *X3* and need not be computed again for *X3* if its value is saved.

8.3.1   Computing Available Expressions

Finding available expressions is similar to finding *reaching definitions.* Again we use the variables *In(B), Out(B).* We use the term *A op B* to mean any expression, even one which has more than one *op,* as in *A + BB * 12.*

Transfer Function Rules

For available expressions, the variables *Kill(B)* and *Gen(B)* are defined as follows:

```
Kill(B) = {the expressions X op Y in the program such
           that X or Y is defined in B},
```

that is, X or Y occurs on the left of an assignment statement or in a read statement.

```
Gen(B) = {the expressions X op Y computed in B, with no
          subsequent definitions of X or Y in B}
```

EXAMPLE 6   Gen and Kill sets for a block B

Consider the following statements in some basic block B

```
A := B + C
X := Y - Z
B := X + Y
X := A * B
```

In Example 6, Gen(B) = {Y – Z, A * B}. Kill(B) = {B + C, X + Y} plus other expressions such as, say, X + Q, since X is on the left-hand side of an assignment in B.

Transfer Equation

We have "rigged" the definition of Gen and Kill for available expressions so that the equation for Out is the same as that for reaching definitions

```
Out(B) = (In(B) - Kill(B)) ∪ Gen(B)
```

Confluence Rule

An expression is available at a point only if it is computed on all preceding paths:

```
In(B) = ∩ Out(P)
       P ∈ Pred(B)
```

We initialize In (start) = φ even though it may have predecessors.

Solving the Equations

This time we want the largest solution since we don't want to rule out an expression unless we find a path along which it is unavailable. Thus, we will initialize the *In* and *Out* sets to make every expression available and then eliminate expressions that are not readily available. Here, we throw things out (via intersection) the way reaching definitions threw things in (via union).

Algorithm
Available Expressions
```
In(Start) = φ
Out(Start) = Gen(Start)
FOR B ≠ Start DO
```

```
    In(B) = All Expressions in program
    Out(B) = (In(B) - Kill(B)) ∪ Gen(B)
ENDFOR
WHILE there are changes DO
    FOR B ≠ Start DO
      In(B) = ∩ Out(P)
          P ∈ Pred(B)
      Out(B) = (In(B) - Kill(B)) ∪ Gen(B)
    ENDFOR
ENDWHILE
```

EXAMPLE 7   Computing available expressions

Consider an expanded version of Example 5:

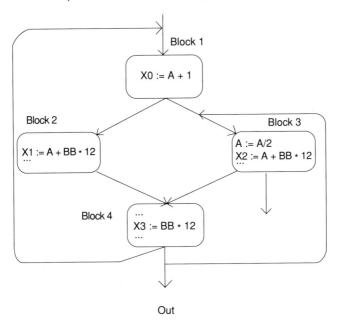

Out

Computing Gen and Kill for each block:

```
Gen(Block1) = {A + 1}                     Kill(Block1) = φ
Gen(Block2) = {BB * 12, A + BB * 12}  Kill(Block2) = φ
Gen(Block3) = {BB * 12, A + BB * 12}  Kill(Block3) =
Gen(Block4) = {BB * 12}                      {A/2, A + 1, A + BB * 12}
                                          Kill(Block4) = φ
```

We compute available expressions using the algorithm:

In(Block 1) = φ
Out(Block 1) = {A +1}

For B ≠ Start. . .

In(Block 2) = {A + 1, BB * 12, A + BB * 12, A/2}
Out(Block 2) = {A + 1, BB * 12, A + BB * 12, A/2}

In(Block 3) = {A + 1, BB * 12, A + BB * 12, A/2}
Out(Block 3) = {BB * 12, A + BB * 12}

In(Block4) = {A + 1, BB * 12, A + BB * 12, A/2}
Out(Block 4) = {A + 1, BB * 12, A + BB * 12, A/2}

WHILE Loop, Iteration 1. . .
                                        WHILE Loop, Iteration 2. . .
In(Block 2) = {A + 1}   In(Block 2) = {A + 1}
Out(Block 2) = {A + 1, BB * 12, A + BB * 12}   Out(Block 2) = {A + 1, BB * 12, A + BB * 12}

In(Block 3) = {A + 1}   In(Block 3) = φ
Out(Block 3) = {BB * 12, A + BB * 12}   Out(Block 3) = {A/2, BB * 12, A + BB * 12}

In(Block 4) = {BB * 12, A + BB * 12}   In(Block 4) = {BB * 12, A + BB * 12}
Out(Block 4) = {BB * 12, A + BB * 12}   Out(Block 4) = {BB * 12, A + BB * 12}

WHILE Loop, Iteration 3. . .
In(Block 2) = {A + 1}
Out(Block 2) = {A + 1, BB * 12, A + BB * 12}

In(Block 3) = φ
Out(Block 3) = {A/2, BB * 12, A + BB * 12}

In(Block 4) = {BB * 12, A + BB * 12}
Out(Block 4) = {BB * 12, A + BB * 12}

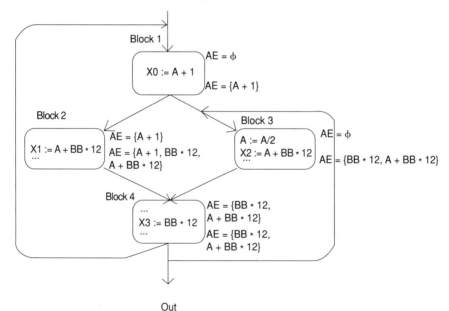

Out

In Example 7, the third iteration of the WHILE loop is the same as the second iteration, so the process terminates.

8.3.2 Use of Available Expressions

Available expressions eliminate recomputations. For example, suppose $In(B)$ contains an expression A op B as does B_4 ($BB * 12$) in Example 7, that is, A op B is available at the beginning of the block as is $BB * 12$ at the beginning of block B_4. Suppose, further, that A op B is used in B (before A or B is redefined). Then we can avoid recomputing A op B in the following way:

1. Find all definitions that reach B and have A op B on the right-hand side.
2. Create a new variable T to hold the value of A op B.
3. Replace each definition $Z := A$ op B from (1) by

```
T := A op B
Z := T
```

4. Replace all uses $Q := A$ op B by $Q := T$.

Example 8 shows this for the program of Example 7 and for the expressions $BB * 12$ and $A + BB * 12$.

EXAMPLE 8 Using an available expressions

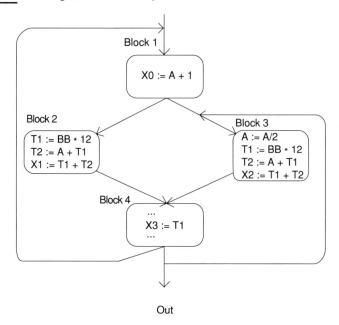

Out

The reader may notice that $BB * 12$ can actually be computed once (in block 1) rather than twice (in block 2 and block 3). This last improvement will be made in Section 6.

8.4   Live Variables

Live variables at a program point P are those for which there is a subsequent *use* before a redefinition.

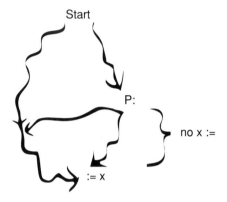

Figure 2

We compute live variables for a number of reasons. If there is a definition not followed by a *use,* then we may want to issue a warning message to the programmer.

Even if there is no definition at a program point P, we may want to keep track of what variables are live to know which ones to keep in registers. If the variable is not to be kept in a register, we may want to store it to reuse the register, but if the variable is not live, we do not need to store it; that is, the code generator does not need to emit a store instruction.

Formally, we define a variable to be *live* at some point in the program if there is some path through the flow graph from that point along which we shall encounter a use of that variable before any redefinition; otherwise, the variable is *dead*.

8.4.1   Equations for Live Variable Analysis

The equations for live variables resemble those for *reaching definitions* except that the data "flows backwards" from the *Out's* to the *In's* rather than from the *In's* to the *Out's*. Note that *In* still refers to the "top" of a block and *Out* to the "bottom", with "top" referring to the part of a block where there is the head of an arrow, and "bottom" meaning a tail.

Transfer Equation

New information transfers from the end to the beginning of a block. We define *Gen* and *Kill,* however, as follows:

```
Kill(B) : {variables defined in B}
Gen(B) : {variables used before a redefinition in B}

  In(B) = (Out(B) − Kill(B)) ∪ Gen(B)
```

Confluence Rule

The confluence rules for backwards flow are really "divergence rules".

```
Out(B) = ∪ In(S)
        S ∈ Succ(B)
```

8.4.2 Algorithm for Computing Live Variables

This time, we once again want the smallest solution—we don't say a variable is live unless we actually find a path along which it is used before being redefined.

Thus, we start by assuming nothing is live on exit from any block. The process stops because we are only adding variables to the sets (and there are a finite number of variables).

Algorithm
Live Variable Analysis
```
FOR all blocks B DO
  In(B) = Gen(B)
ENDFOR
WHILE there are changes DO
  FOR each block B DO
    Out(B) = ∪ In(S)
            S ∈ Succ(B)
    In(B) = (Out(B) − Kill(B)) ∪ Gen(B)
  ENDFOR
ENDWHILE
```

EXAMPLE 9 Live variable analysis

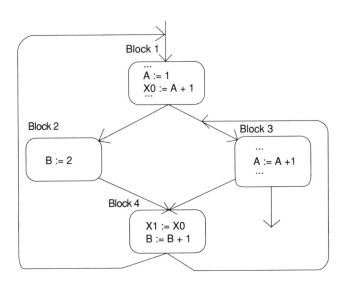

```
Gen(Block1) = φ            Kill(Block1) = {A, X0}
Gen(Block2) = φ            Kill(Block2) = {B}
Gen(Block3) = {A}          Kill(Block3) = {A}
Gen(Block4) = {X0, B}      Kill(Block4) = {X1, B}
```

FOR Loop ...

```
In(Block1) = φ
In(Block2) = φ
In(Block3) = {A}
In(Block4) = {X0, B}
```

WHILE, Iteration 1:

```
Out(Block1) = {A}           In(Block1) = φ
Out(Block2) = {X0, B}       In(Block2) = {X0}
Out(Block3) = {X0, B}       In(Block3) = {X0, B, A}
Out(Block4) = {X0, B, A}    In(Block4) = {X0, B, A}
```

WHILE, Iteration 2:

```
Out(Block1) = {X0, B, A}    In(Block1) = {B}
Out(Block2) = {X0, B, A}    In(Block2) = {X0, A}
Out(Block3) = {X0, B, A}    In(Block3) = {X0, B, A}
Out(Block4) = {X0, B, A}    In(Block4) = {X0, B, A}
```

WHILE, Iteration 3:

```
Out(Block1) = {X0, B, A}    In(Block1) = {B}
Out(Block2) = {X0, B, A}    In(Block2) = {X0, A}
Out(Block3) = {X0, B, A}    In(Block3) = {X0, B, A}
Out(Block4) = {X0, B, A}    In(Block4) = {X0, B, A}
```

Iteration 3 of the WHILE loop is the same as iteration 2; thus we are done.

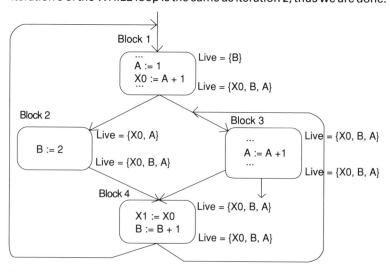

8.4.3 Data Structures for Live Variables

The ideas are the same as for reaching definitions. We can identify variables with positions in a bit vector, using a table of pointers (perhaps to the symbol table) to make the association.

8.5 Reached Uses

Reached uses is a similar problem to live variable analysis.

A *Use* of A is *reached* from the assignment statement A := if there is some path from the assignment to the use along which A is not redefined.

EXAMPLE 10 Reached use

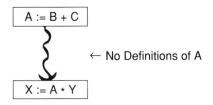

We can detect useless assignments: they are those assignments with no reached uses.

To find the equations for *reached uses,* note that the last definition of A in a block B reaches what the end of block B reaches, plus subsequent uses of A within B. Prior definitions of A *within* B reach only their uses within B.

Equations for Reached Uses

The domain is somewhat different here: the set of pairs consisting of a statement S and a variable A appearing on the right of S.

```
Kill(B) = {(S,A) | S not in B and B contains an
                   assignment to A}
Gen(B) = {(S,A) | S ∈ B, A on right-hand side of S, and
                  no definitions of A prior to S in B}
```

Transfer Equation

```
In(B) = (Out(B) − Kill(B)) ∪ Gen(B)
```

Confluence Equation

```
Out(B) = ∪ In(S)
         S ∈ Succ(B)
```

The algorithm is essentially the same as that for live variables; that is, we assume nothing is reached, and apply the equations. The result is the smallest solution since a *use* is *reached* only if we can really find a path to it.

8.6   Very Busy Expressions

An expression *A op B* is *very busy* at a point *p* if along *every* path from *p* there is an expression *A op B* before a redefinition of either *A* or *B*.

If an expression is very busy at program point *p*, it makes sense to compute it there. This is often termed *code hoisting* and it saves *space* although it doesn't necessarily save *time*.

But it is interesting as a fourth type of data flow analysis problem: backwards flow and intersection confluence.

8.6.1   Equations for Very Busy Expressions

```
Kill(B) = {X op Y | either X or Y defined before
                use of X op Y in B}
Gen(B) = {X op Y | X op Y used in B before any
                definition of X or Y}
```

Transfer Equation

```
In(B) = (Out(B) − Kill(B)) ∪ Gen(B)
```

Confluence Equation

```
Out(B) = ∩ In(S)
       S ∈ Succ(B)
```

Algorithm for Computing Very Busy Expressions

We want to avoid considering *X op Y* as *very busy* just because neither *X* nor *Y* is redefined. To do this, we introduce a dummy block D such that

```
Kill(D) = all expressions
Gen(D) = none
```

and we let D be a successor of all blocks that have the program end as a possible successor.

Algorithm
Very Busy Expressions
```
FOR each block B DO
  Out(B) := all expressions
  In(B) := (Out(B) − Kill(B)) ∪ Gen(B))

END
WHILE there are changes DO
  FOR each block B DO
  Out(B) = ∩ In(S)
         S ∈ Succ(B)

  In(B) = (Out(B) − Kill(B)) ∪ Gen(B)
ENDFOR
ENDWHILE
```

EXAMPLE 11   Computing very busy expressions

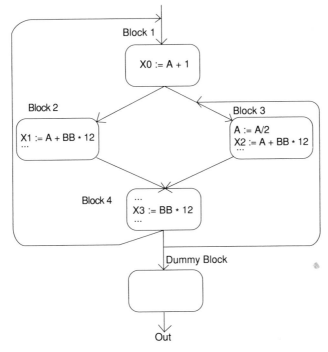

Gen(Block1) = {A + 1}   Kill(Block1) = φ
Gen(Block2) = {BB * 12, A + BB * 12}   Kill(Block2) = φ
Gen(Block3) = {A/2, BB * 12}   Kill(Block3) =
                                                    {A + BB * 12}
Gen(Block4) = {BB * 12}   Kill(Block4) = φ
Gen(D)   = φ   Kill(D) =
                                             {A + 1, A/2, BB * 12,
                                                    A + BB * 12}

FOR Loop ...

Out(Block1) = {A + 1, A/2, BB * 12, A + BB * 12}
In(Block1) = {A + 1, A/2, BB * 12, A + BB * 12}
Out(Block2) = {A + 1, A/2, BB * 12, A + BB * 12}
In(Block2) = {A + 1, A/2, BB * 12, A + BB * 12}
Out(Block3) = {A + 1, A/2, BB * 12, A + .BB * 12}
In(Block3) = {A + 1, A/2, BB * 12}
Out(Block4) = {A + 1, A/2, BB * 12, A + BB * 12}
In(Block4) = {A + 1, A/2, BB * 12, A + BB * 12}
Out(D)   = {A + 1, A/2, BB * 12, A + BB * 12}
In(D)   = φ

WHILE Loop Iteration 1 ...

Out(Block1) = {A + 1, A/2, BB * 12}
In(Block1) = {A + 1, A/2, BB * 12}

```
Out(Block2) = {A + 1, A/2, BB * 12, A + BB * 12}
In(Block2)  = {A + 1, A/2, BB * 12, A + BB * 12}
Out(Block3) = {A + 1, A/2, BB * 12, A + BB * 12}
In(Block3)  = {A + 1, A/2, BB * 12}
Out(Block4) = φ
In(Block4)  = {BB * 12}
Out(D)      = φ
In(D)       = φ
```

WHILE Loop Iteration 2 ...

```
Out(Block1) = {A + 1, A/2, BB * 12}
In(Block1)  = {A + 1, A/2, BB * 12}
Out(Block2) = {BB * 12}
In(Block2)  = {BB * 12, A + BB * 12}
Out(Block3) = {BB * 12}
In(Block3)  = {A/2, BB * 12}
Out(Block4) = φ
In(Block4)  = {BB * 12}
Out(D)      = φ
In(D)       = φ
```

WHILE Loop Iteration 3 ...

```
Out(Block1) = {BB * 12}
In(Block1)  = {A + 1, BB * 12}
Out(Block2) = {BB * 12}
In(Block2)  = {BB * 12, A + BB * 12}
Out(Block3) = {BB * 12}
In(Block3)  = {A/2, BB * 12}
Out(Block4) = φ
In(Block4)  = {BB * 12}
Out(D)      = φ
In(D)       = φ
```

WHILE Loop Iteration 4 ...

```
Out(Block1) = {BB * 12}
In(Block1)  = {A + 1, BB * 12}
Out(Block2) = {BB * 12}
In(Block2)  = {BB * 12, A + BB * 12}
Out(Block3) = {BB * 12}
In(Block3)  = {A/2, BB * 12}
Out(Block4) = φ
In(Block4)  = {BB * 12}
Out(D)      = φ
In(D)       = φ
```

Iteration 4 is the same as iteration 3; thus, we are done.

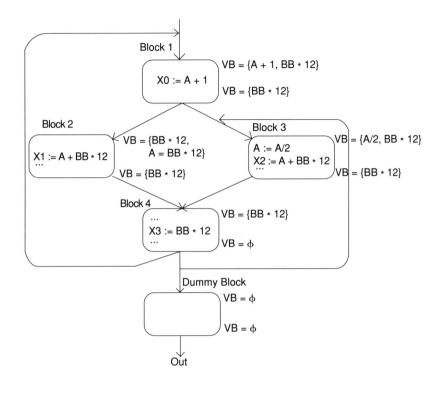

8.7 High-Level Data Flow Analysis

We can perform data flow analysis on a tree when the tree is known to represent the program flow (e.g., no multiple entries and exits from loops, no GOTO's, etc.).

The following live variable analysis is described by Babich and Jazayeri (1978a). They compute dead variables and available expressions. We will discuss dead variables. Exercise 9 asks the reader to write the equations for available expressions and reaching definitions.

A variable is defined as *dead* at a point in a program if its value will not be used after control leaves that point.

The following (ambiguous) grammar will be used:

```
Statement → Statement₁ Statement₂
Statement → IF Expression THEN Statement₁ ELSE
                                             Statement₂
Statement → WHILE Expression DO Statement
Statement → Label : Statement
Statement → GOTO Statement
Statement → Assignment
Statement → ReadStatement
Statement → WriteStatement
```

The following notation will be used for the tree nodes:

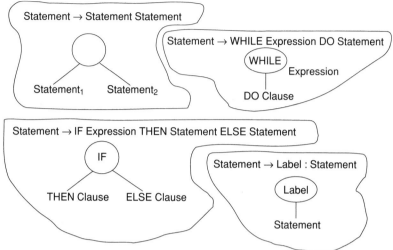

Four Boolean attributes, *Kill, Gen, DeadAtBeginning* and *DeadAtEnd,* will be associated with each of these nodes. For simplicity, only one variable will be analyzed. Exercise 7 asks the reader to extend this for more than one variable. The equations will reflect the following:

```
Statement.DeadAtBeginning := True if the variable is
                DEAD at the beginning of Statement.
Statement.DeadAtEnd := True if the variable is DEAD
                        at the end of Statement.
Statement.Kill := True if the variable is assigned a
                        value in Statement.
Statement.Used := True if the variable is used and
    not assigned in Statement or else used in Statement
                before being assigned in Statement.
```

We will define these first two more precisely below. The algorithm will iterate because none of the methods we have developed so far will work (see Exercise 6).

Since deadness at a point is inherently a property of the portion of the program that comes *after* that point, we need to have scanned the portion of the tree to the right of that node. Thus, we scan the tree from *right* to *left*.

The attributes *DeadAtBeginning* and *DeadAtEnd* are defined as follows:

For Assignment, Read, and Write statements:

```
Statement.DeadAtBeginning := NOT(Statement.Used)
                        AND (Statement.Kill |
                            Statement.DeadAtEnd)
```

For Statement → Statement$_1$ Statement$_2$, we note that we want to start with the value of Statement.*DeadAtEnd* and compute Statement.*DeadAtBeginning* and that the *end* of Statement$_1$ is also the *beginning* of Statement$_2$. Therefore,

```
Statement₂.DeadAtEnd := Statement.DeadAtBeginning
```

and since the *end* of Statement$_1$ is also the *beginning* of Statement$_2$,

```
Statement₁.DeadAtEnd := Statement₂.DeadAtBeginning
```

The beginning of Statement$_1$ is the same point as the beginning of Statement, so:

```
Statement.DeadAtBeginning := Statement₁.DeadAtBeginning
```

The equations for IF statements and WHILE statements are similar. The attribute grammar is:

```
(1) Statement → Statement₁ Statement₂
    (i) Statement₂.DeadAtEnd := Statement.DeadAtBeginning
    (ii) Statement₁.DeadAtEnd := Statement₂.DeadAtBeginnin
    (iii) Statement₁.DeadAtEnd := Statement₂.DeadAtBeginning

(2) Statement → IF Expression THEN Statement₁ ELSE Statement₂
    (i) Statement₂.DeadAtEnd := Statement.DeadAtEnd
    (ii) Statement₁.DeadAtEnd := Statement.DeadAtEnd
    (iii) Statement.DeadAtBeginning := NOT (Expression.Used)
          AND (Statement₁.DeadAtBeginning AND Statement₂.
          DeadAtBeginning)

(3) Statement → WHILE Expression DO Statement
    (i) Statement.DeadAtEnd := NOT (Expression.Used) AND
        (Statement.DeadAtEnd AND Statement₁.DeadAtBeginning)
    (ii) Statement.DeadAtBeginning := NOT (Expression.Used) AND
         (Statement.DeadAtEnd  AND Statement₁.DeadAtBeginning)

(4) Statement → Label : Statement
    (i) Statement₁.DeadAtEnd := Statement.DeadAtEnd
    (ii) Statement.DeadAtBeginning := Statement₁.DeadAtBegin-
         ning

(5) Statement → GOTO Statement
    (i) Statement.DeadAtBeginning := TargetStatement.DeadAt-
        Beginning

(6) Statement → Assignment | ReadStatement | WriteStatement
    (i) Statement.DeadAtBeginning := NOT (Statement.Used) AND
    (Statement.Kill | Statement.DeadAtEnd)
```

For the WHILE loop the rules for Statement$_1$.*DeadAtEnd* and Statement.*DeadAt-Beginning* are the same because an exit from the body of a WHILE loop is followed by a branch back to reenter the loop.

It may be necessary to compute the attributes at a node more than once before the correct values are computed. The (recursive) algorithm to compute attribute values for each statement is:

Algorithm
Dead (Statement)
```
BEGIn {Dead}
FOR each component of Statement,
    in right to left order,
BEGIn
  Compute Component.DeadAtEnd
  Call DEAD(Component)
END
Compute Statement.DeadAtBeginning
END {Dead}
```

The values for *DeadAtEnd* and *DeadAtBeginning* are saved in the tree as they are computed. Thus each tree node contains at least the following information: (1) node type (compound, IF, WHILE, etc.), (2) the values of *DeadAtEnd* and *DeadAtBeginning*, (3) assorted pointers to other nodes, describing the position of the node in the tree and (4) values of *Used* and *Kill* where needed.

In a pass over the tree, attributes whose values are needed will usually be computed before they are used. In two cases, however, this will not be true. The first case is backward GOTO's since the right to left scan will not have computed the right-hand side of the semantic function. The second case is for WHILE statements since to find *DeadAtEnd*, we need *DeadAtBeginning*, which isn't know because Statement$_1$ hasn't been analyzed yet. Because of these two cases, we initialize these attributes to True.

The evaluation algorithm iterates until no attribute value changes.

Algorithm
Dead(Tree)
```
While there are changes to any attribute value DO
  Initialize attributes to True
  BEGIn
    Store Root.DeadAtEnd and Call Dead(Root)
    Store any changed values
  END
```

Example 12 shows a program and the values after two passes over the tree, analyzing the attribute values for the variable *A*.

EXAMPLE 12   High-level data flow analysis example

```
Read A
WHILE B ≠ 0 DO
```

```
BEGIn
   Write A
   WHILE A < 5 DO
     BEGIn
       A := A + 1
       Write A
       B := A
     END
   Read(A)
END
```

Pass 0 (Initializing Attributes to True):

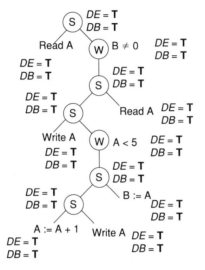

Pass 1:

Example 12 shows the initialization pass and pass 1 of the evaluation.
The reader is asked to perform the remaining passes in Exercise 8.

8.8   Interprocedural Data Flow Analysis

The preceding sections have discussed *intraprocedural* data flow analysis, that is,
data flow analysis within a procedure. *Interprocedural* data flow analysis discusses
the same issues, but with intervening function or procedure calls. This is shown
below, where we might ask if expression $x + Op\ y$ is available. If function f does not
modify either x or $y,$ then it will be available.

```
A : X + Y
. . .
Y := f(A)
. . .
B := X + Y
```

One method is to assume a worst case: no expressions will be available after a subprogram call, no variables are live, etc.

To perform a more accurate interprocedural data flow analysis, we need to calculate the *call* chain, that is, what subprograms are called within a subprogram.

Interprocedural analysis often involves finding *aliases*. A variable X is an *alias* of
a variable Y if X and Y are different names for the same memory location. *Reference*
parameters are an example of aliasing, as are assigning the value of one pointer to
another. Thus, changing one of the variables effectively changes the other.

For languages which require explicit declaration of global variables and reference
parameters, it may be reasonable to perform an interprocedural analysis. Reference
parameters and globals which are changed in the procedure may be identified via
Gen and Kill sets.

Changes to any element of an array are usually recorded as having changed the
entire array since it may be impossible to tell at compile time which element will be
changed.

8.9   Summary

This chapter discussed data flow problems, at first on the low-level control flow
graph and then on an abstract syntax tree representation. Data flow problems can be
divided into two types: backwards flow problems and forward flow problems. They
can also be partitioned into problems whose confluence rules use union and those
which use intersection. The following figure shows the five problems discussed in
this chapter in these categories:

Four Data Flow Analysis Categories

	Some (Any) $\cup$	**All** (Every) $\cap$
Forward (Use Predecessors)	*Reaching Definitions* Which definitions reach a point by *some* path?	*Available Expressions* Which expressions are available on *all* paths to a point?
Backwards (Use Successors)	*Live Variables Reached uses* Which variables have a subsequent use on *some* path?	*Very Busy Expressions* Which expressions are used (computed) on all paths subsequent to a point?

We will use data flow analysis in the next chapter when we discuss specific examples and specific optimization categories.

In Chapter 12, we will look at data flow analysis again when we discuss incremental compiling.

8.10   Related Reading

Babich, W. A. & M. Jazayeri. 1978a. The Methods of Attributes for Data Flow Analysis, Part I. Exhaustive Analysis, *Acta Informatica*, 10:245–264.
Contains a sample attribute grammar for performing data flow analysis on a tree.

Babich, W. A. & M. Jazayeri. 1978b. The Methods of Attributes for Data Flow Analysis, Part II. Demand Analysis, *Acta Informatica*, 10:265–272.

Barry, R. 1988. An Attribute Grammar for Building Intraprocedural Data Dependence Graphs, Master's Thesis, Worcester, MA: Worcester Polytechnic Institute, CS Dept.
Same as the preceding except the data flow information is computed when needed by the optimizer.

Cooper, K., K. Kennedy, and L. Torczon. 1986. The Impact of Interprocedural Analysis and Optimization in the R^n Programming Environment, *ACM Transactions on Programming Languages and Systems*, 8(4):491–523.

Marlowe, T. J. and B. G. Ryder. 1989. Properties of Data Flow Frameworks: A Unified Model, *Acta Informatica*.

Mintz, R. J., G. A. Fishewe Jr., and M. Sharir. 1979. *The Design of a Global Optimizer*, SIGPLAN Conference on Compiler Construction, 226–234.

Rosen, B. 1977. High-Level Data Flow Analysis, *CACM*, 20(10):712–724.

Ryder, B. G. and M. C. Paull. 1986. Elimination Algorithms for Data Flow Analysis, *ACM Computing Surveys*, 18(3):277–316.

Sacks, R. 1989. Detecting Interprocedural Parallelism During Semantic Analysis, Master's thesis, Worcester, MA: Worcester Polytechnic Institute, CS Dept.

Sequential programs are analyzed to find procedures which may be performed in parallel.

Sharir, M. 1980. Structural Analysis: A New Approach to Flow Analysis in Optimizing Compilers, *Computer Languages*, 5:141–153

Tarjan, R. E. 1981. Fast Algorithms for Solving Path Problems, *Journal of the ACM*, 27(3):594–614.

EXERCISES

1. Change the following example so that the expression $X + Y$ is available
   (a) At the end of block 2
   (b) At the beginning of block 3

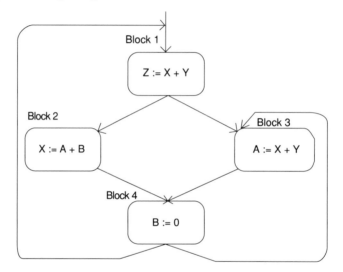

2. The following is the control flow graph for the example from the beginning of Chapter 7:

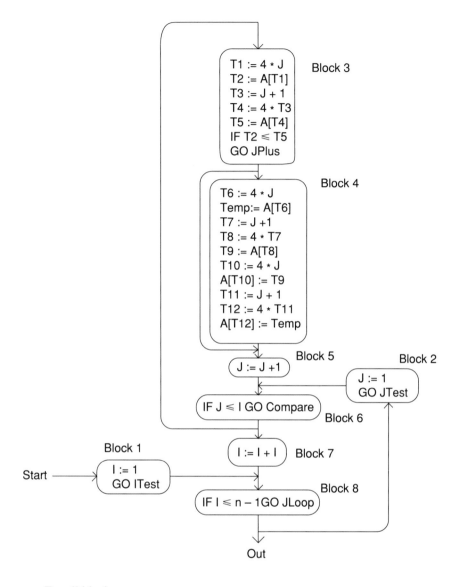

For all blocks, compute
(a) Reaching definitions
(b) Live variables
(c) Available expressions
(d) Reached uses
(e) Very busy expressions

3. There may really be more available expressions than the definition for available expressions finds. Find such a case.

4. Show how the procedure call $P(x,x)$ might create aliases.

5. Using the method of Section 8.7, define equations for available expression analysis (Babich and Jazayeri, 1978a).

6. Define Gen and Kill sets for interprocedural analysis of
   (a) Live variables
   (b) Available expressions

7. The grammar of Section 8.7 fails to be an attribute grammar as defined in Chapter 6 for two reasons. What are they?

8. By using set-valued equations, extend the equations of Section 8.7 to include all the variables in a program. Perform the data flow analysis for Example 12 using these equations.

9. For Example 12:
   (a) Show the step by step details of pass 1.
   (b) Show the remaining passes.

10. Using Section 8.7 as a model, write the equations for
    (a) Available expressions
    (b) Reaching definitions

   For each, perform the analysis on the program of Example 12.

9

Optimization: Code Improvement

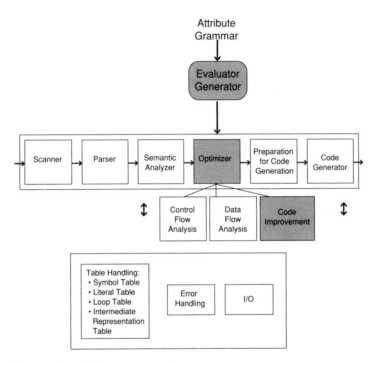

9.0 Introduction

This chapter uses the material of the last two chapters to describe program improvements. We divide optimizations into three categories: (i) local optimizations, (ii) global optimizations and (iii) loop optimizations. Chapter 10 discusses another way to improve programs by allocating registers creatively. The last program improvement, *peephole* optimization, which is performed after code is selected, is also discussed in Chapter 10.

We also include two examples, one which optimizes on the control flow graph and one which optimizes at a higher level on the abstract syntax tree.

We show much of the intermediate representation in this chapter as quadruples; they are much easier to read than abstract syntax trees. This method suffers from the *Heisenberg Uncertainty Principle* (which the reader may remember from chemistry or physics); it affects the very code we are trying to improve. Quadruples introduce many temporary variables which we will eliminate when possible. Otherwise, the same information can be discovered in trees as in three-address code. Throughout this chapter, we use the term *optimization*, knowing that we really mean *improvement*.

9.1   Local Optimizations

Local optimizations improve code *within* basic blocks. Although the separation is somewhat hazy, we won't include as a local optimization anything that moves code outside a block or uses information from outside a block.

In a sense, this category is redundant. Almost all local optimizations have their global counterpart. The method of detection is often different, however.

9.1.1   Local Common Subexpression Elimination

Local common subexpressions are detected automatically when a DAG is created. They can also be detected by using the methods of Chapter 8, which find common subexpressions globally.

EXAMPLE 1   Local common subexpression elimination

```
T1 := BB * 12              T1 := BB * 12
T2 := A + T1               T2 := A + T1
X1 := T1          →        X1 := T1
T3 := BB * 12              T4 := A/2
T4 := A/2                  T5 := T4 + T1
T5 := T4 + T3              X2 := T5
X2 := T5
```

9.1.2   Local Strength Reduction

Computers add faster than they multiply, multiply faster than they raise to powers, etc. Replacing an operator by its definition is termed *strength reduction*. For example, if B is a compile-time constant

```
A * B = A + A + A (B times)
```

When one of the factors is a small integer such as 2, it is worth replacing the operator.

EXAMPLE 2   Local strength reduction

```
T1 := 2 * A → T1 := A + A
```

Example 2 replaces a multiplication by 2 with an addition. If the factor is not a small number like 2, then sometimes a combination of multiplications and shifts may be done (see Exercise 1).

9.1.3 Local Constant Propagation and Folding

Constants are produced, not only by the programmer, but also by the compiler. The programmer may initialize a variable to be 1, using this as both a loop counter and as an array index. Then, in allocating space for the array, the compiler may multiply such elements by 4 to indicate that they are to use four bytes of storage. We show such a situation in Example 3.

EXAMPLE 3   Local constant propagation

```
I := 2                      I := 2
...              →          ...
T1 := 4 * I                 T1:= 4 * 2
```

A related optimization computes constant expressions at compile-time rather than generating code to perform the optimization.

EXAMPLE 4   Constant folding

```
I := 2                      I := 2
...              →          ...
T1 := 4 * 2                 T1 := 8
```

Constant folding is sometimes called constant *computation.* It can require a little more alertness on the part of the compiler, as shown in Example 5.

EXAMPLE 5   Constant folding

```
I := 2 * I        →      I:= 8 * I
(no reference to I)
I := 4 * I
```

In Example 5, I has been modified twice.

9.1.4 Algebraic Identities

An algebraic identity performs a substitution using algebraic laws. We list a few:

```
1. X := A + 0             →   X := A
2. X := 1 * A             →   X := A
3. Constant * Symbol  →   Symbol * Constant
```

Algebraic substitution can substitute one expression in a basic block with another, as shown in Example 6.

EXAMPLE 6   Algebraic substitution

```
T1 := 4 * J - 1        T1 := 4 * J - 1
...              →      ...
T7 := T1 + 1           T7 := 4 * J
```

9.2   Loop Optimizations

Most programs spend the majority of their time in loops. The payoff in optimizing loops is, on the average, greater than any other optimizations.

In Chapter 7, we discussed how to identify a loop. We use that here when performing loop optimizations.

In particular, there is a useful property of loops: two *natural* loops are either disjoint (except for the header) or one is nested within the other.

Two loops with the same header should probably be merged into one:

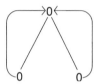

We will use the property that two natural loops are either nested or disjoint for some loop optimizations. The two most common optimizations are detection and movement of invariant code and induction variable elimination. Other optimizations optimize special loop forms such as loops which make changes to array elements one by one or pairs of loops with the same execution conditions.

9.2.1   Loop-Invariant Computations and Code Motion

Loop-invariant statements are those statements within a loop which produce the same value each time the loop is executed. We identify them and then move them outside the loop.

Example 7 shows a control flow graph and a loop-invariant statement.

EXAMPLE 7   Loop invariants

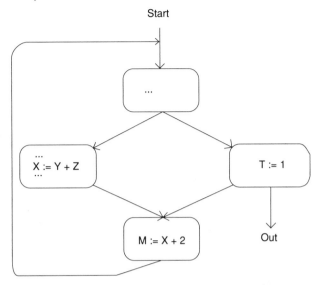

In Example 7, $T := 1$ is loop-invariant (presuming no assignment to T in the header) and may be moved outside the loop. The statement $X := Y + Z$ is not loop invariant (why?).

Finding Loop-Invariant Statements

If all definitions of y and z in $x := y \; op \; z$ are outside the loop, then the statement is invariant. These statements can be found in one pass through the loop. There may be more, however, since any statements using variables in loop-invariant statements are also loop-invariant. The method is to iterate until no more are found.

EXAMPLE 8   Finding loop invariants

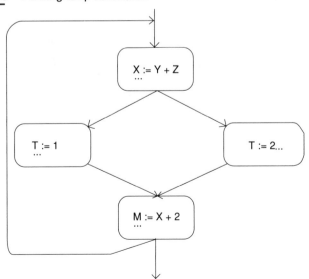

The definitions of *Y* and *Z* reaching *X := Y + Z* are outside the loop. This statement is then invariant. On a second pass, *M := X + 2* can be found to be loop-invariant. Once loop-invariant statements have been found, they are moved. One way to do this is to create a *preheader*.

Preheaders

For each loop, create a new block, which has only the header as a successor. This is called a preheader and is not part of the loop. It is used to hold statements moved out of the loop. Here, these are the loop-invariant statements. In the next section, the preheader will be used to hold initializations for the induction variables.

Code Motion Algorithm

If a statement is loop-invariant, it is moved to the preheader *provided* (1) the movement does not change what the program computes and (2) the program does not slow up.

Algorithm
Loop-Invariant Code Motion

Given the nodes in a loop, compute the definitions reaching the header and dominators.
Find the loop-invariant statements.
Find the exits of the loop: the nodes with a successor outside the loop.
Select for code motion those statements that:

> (i) are loop-invariant and
> (ii) are in blocks that dominate exits and
> (iii) are in blocks that dominate all blocks in the loop which use
> their computed values and
> (iv) assign to variables not assigned to elsewhere in loop

Perform a depth-first search of the loop. Visit each block in depth-first order, moving all statements selected above to the preheader.

The last step preserves the execution order.

EXAMPLE 9 Loop-invariant code motion

Example 9a *Moving the loop-invariant statement T := 1*

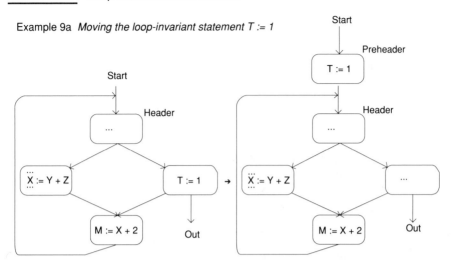

Example 9b *Moving the loop-invariant statement M := X + Z and X := Y + Z*

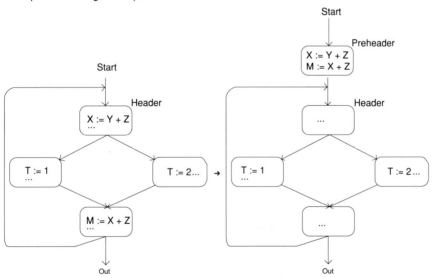

This example shows the loop-invariant statements of the preceding examples moved to a preheader in the right graphs.

Moving statements to the preheader may cause the program to slow down if the loop is never entered. The criterion that the loop never slow down may be enforced by executing the statements in the preheader only if the loop is executed.

Taking this one step further, the condition:

```
WHILE Condition DO Statements
```

becomes

```
IF Condition
  THEN Preheader
  REPEAT
    Statements
  UNTIL NOT Condition
ENDIF
```

Now the preheader is executed only if the loop is entered.

9.2.2   Induction Variable Detection and Elimination

An induction variable is a variable whose value on each loop iteration is a linear function of the iteration index. When such variables and the expressions they compute are found, often the variable itself can be eliminated or a strength reduction can be performed.

EXAMPLE 10   Induction variable

```
J := 0
FOR I := 1 to N DO
   . . .
   J := J + 1
   K := 2 * J
   M := 3 * K
   . . .
   A[M] :=
ENDFOR
```

J, K, and *M* are all induction variables. (The loop index, *I,* is trivially an induction variable.)

EXAMPLE 11   More induction variables

```
t := b * c
FOR i := 1 TO 10000 DO
  BEGIN
    a := t
    d := i * 3
    . . .
  END
    . . .
```

d is an induction variable.

The most common induction variables are those which result from indexing elements of an array. Multiplications of the index are created when an array takes more than one byte or when the offset is computed for multidimensional arrays.

Induction Variables

We find induction variables incrementally. A *basic induction variable* is a variable X whose only assignments within the loop are of the form:

```
X := X + C
X := X - C
```

where C is a constant or a loop-invariant variable. In Example 10, I and J are basic induction variables.

We define an *induction variable, recursively,* to be a basic induction variable or one which is a linear function of some induction variable. In Example 10, K is an induction variable since K is a linear function of J. M is an induction variable since $M := 3 * K = 3 * (2 * J) = 6 * J$. The expressions $J + 1, 2 * J$, and $3 * K$ are called induction expressions.

Finding Induction Variables

After reaching definitions find all definitions of Y and Z in $X := Y \ op \ Z$ which reach the beginning of the loop, basic induction variables can be found by a simple scan of the loop. To find other induction variables, we find variables, W, such that

```
W := A * X + B
```

where A and B are constants or loop invariants, and X is an induction variable. These can be found by iterating through the loop until no more induction variables are found.

In Example 10, the variable J reaches the top of the loop. The statement $J := J + 1$ satisfies the definition of a basic induction variable. The other statements will be found on successive visits through the loop.

9.2.3 Strength Reduction

Although strength reduction is, strictly speaking, a global optimization, it rarely pays off except in loops.

Consider the multiplication in Example 11. Since d is an induction variable, we can replace the induction expression $i * 3$ by initializing d to its initial value, 3, outside the loop and then adding 3 on each loop iteration. This is shown in Example 12.

EXAMPLE 12   Strength reduction

```
t := b * c                          t := b * c
FOR i:= 1 TO 10000 DO               d := 0
  BEGIN                               FOR i:= 1 TO 10000 DO
    a:= t                   →           BEGIN
    d:= i * 3                             a := t
    . . .                                 d := d + 3
  END                                     . . .
                                        END
```

We have shown the example for a strength reduction of a multiplication to an addition, but other strength reductions may be performed also (see Exercise 7).

We list some other optimizations for loops here, with the exercises exploring how these optimizations would be found from data flow analyses, loop invariants and loop inductions.

9.2.4   Loop Unrolling

Loop unrolling decreases the number of iterations of a loop. Consider the following loop:

```
LOOP I = 1 to 10000 by 1
  A(I) := A(I) + B(I)
ENDLOOP
```

Unrolling by 2 gives

```
LOOP I = 1 to 9999 by 2
  A(I) = A(I) + B(I)
  A(I + 1) = A(I + 1) + B(I + 1)
ENDLOOP
```

The number of instructions *executed* is reduced because the number of increments and tests is halved.

Another example of loop unrolling is:

```
WHILE Condition              WHILE Condition
  A                →           A
ENDWHILE                       IF NOT Condition THEN Exit
                               A
                             ENDLOOP
```

Loop unrolling also exposes instructions for parallel execution since the two statements can be executed at the same time if they are independent (see Chapter 12).

The disadvantage here is that increased instruction space is required.

9.2.5   Loop Jamming (Fusion)

Sometimes two loops may be replaced by one. Consider the following loops:

```
LOOP I := 1 to 100
  A(I) := 0
ENDLOOP
LOOP I := 1 to 100
  B(I) = X(I) + Y
ENDLOOP
```

These two loops can be "fused":

```
LOOP I := 1 to 100
  A(I) = 0
  B(I) = X(I) + Y
ENDLOOP
```

The loop overhead is reduced, resulting in a speed-up in execution, as well as a reduction in code space. Once again, instructions are exposed for parallel execution.

The conditions for performing this optimization are that the loop indices be the same and the computations in one loop cannot depend on the computations in the other loop.

Sometimes loops may be fused when one loop index is a subset of the other:

```
FOR I := 1 TO 10000 DO
          A[I] := 0
FOR J := 1 TO 5000 DO
          B[J] := 0
                ↓

      FOR I := 1 TO 10000 DO
          IF I ≤ 5000 THEN B[I] := 0
          A[I] := 0
```

Here, a test has been added to compute the second loop within the first. The loop must execute many times for this optimization to be worthwhile.

9.2.6   Count up to Zero

This transformation simplifies the termination test (computers often have separate instructions to test for 0):

```
LOOP FOR I := 1 TO N DO          LOOP FOR I := 1 - N TO 0
    ... I ...              →               ... I + N ...
ENDLOOP                          ENDLOOP
```

9.2.7   Unswitching

```
LOOP FOR I := 1 TO 1000
  IF (Test) THEN
    X(I):= A(I) + B(I)
  ELSE
    X(I):= A(I) - B(I)
ENDLOOP
```

Here, the test is performed each time through the loop. The following performs the test once:

```
IF (Test) THEN
  LOOP FOR I := 1 to 1000
    X(I) = A(I) + B(I)
  ENDLOOP
  ELSE
    LOOP FOR I := 1 to 100
      X(I) = A(I) - B(I)
  ENDLOOP
```

The second version here reduces the number of instructions executed, but the code takes more space.

9.2.8   Loop Collapse

Sometimes, as the result of other optimizations, the body of a loop becomes vacuous. It may then be removed:

```
LOOP
ENDLOOP          →          Null
```

9.3   Global Optimizations

Many global optimizations are analogous to local ones, but use data flow analysis to find optimizations between blocks. Even though we include them here, in *global* optimization, their payoff is greater when they also reduce the computations in a loop.

9.3.1   Redundant (Common) Subexpression Elimination

Figure 1 shows an expression *X op Y* which may be computed once on each path and then used.

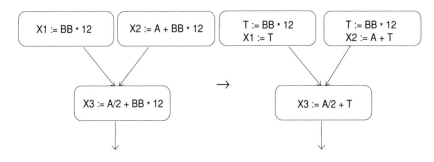

Figure 1

9.3.2   Global Constant Folding and Propagation

From *reaching definitions*, a use-definition chain, *ud-chain*, can be constructed. This is a list of variable definitions linked with their uses. Within a block, a definition is matched to its subsequent use. If there is no definition within the block, then all definitions which reach the block are matched with the use.

The ud-chain may be used for constant propagation.

EXAMPLE 13   Global constant propagation

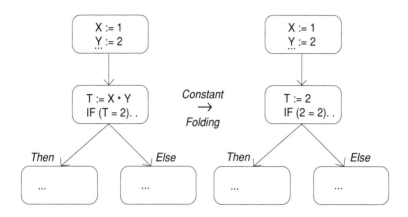

This can be optimized still further with an algebraic substitution and a dead code elimination. The result is shown in Example 14.

9.3.3   Dead Code Elimination

As the result of previous optimizations, both statements and entire blocks may now be unnecessary.

EXAMPLE 14   Dead code elimination on Example 13

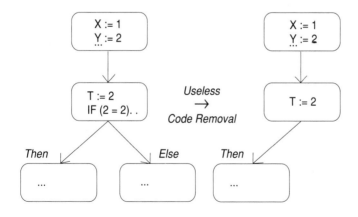

9.3.4   Conditional Pruning

The general cases for Example 14 are:

```
IF True THEN
  A              →          A
ELSE
  B
```

and

```
IF False THEN
  A              →          B
ELSE
  B
```

9.3.5   Conditional Reordering

Sometimes a conditional can be reordered:

```
IF Condition THEN              IF NOT Condition THEN
  Null                  →          A
ELSE A                            ENDIF
ENDIF
```

9.3.6   Assignment Elimination Due to Equality

If it is known via data flow analysis and perhaps other optimizations that *Value(A)* = *Value(B)*, then

```
A := B        →          Null
```

This presumes that *A* and *B* really are the same variable; that is, they are not both needed later.

9.3.7   GOTO Chasing

The following code is often generated by IF-THEN-ELSE statements or CASE statements:

```
    GOTO LabelA                   GOTO LabelB
       ...        →                  ...
LabelA: GOTO LabelB         LabelA: GOTO LabelB
```

9.3.8   Array Temporary Elimination

Computing the offsets for array references is time consuming and may often be eliminated when the value is used:

```
A[I,J] := B * C              T := B * C
    ...              →           ...
A[J,I] := A[I,J] + 1         A[J,I] := T + 1
```

9.4   An Example

In this section, we perform an example which includes many of the optimizations discussed so far:

Consider the algorithm for a Bubblesort from Chapter 7:

```
FOR I := 1 TO N - 1 DO
  FOR J := 1 TO i DO
    IF A[J] > A[J + 1] THEN
      Temp := A[J]
      A[J] := A[J + 1]
      A[J + 1] := Temp
    ENDIF
  ENDFOR
ENDFOR
```

The intermediate representation (shown as quadruples) and the control flow graph are:

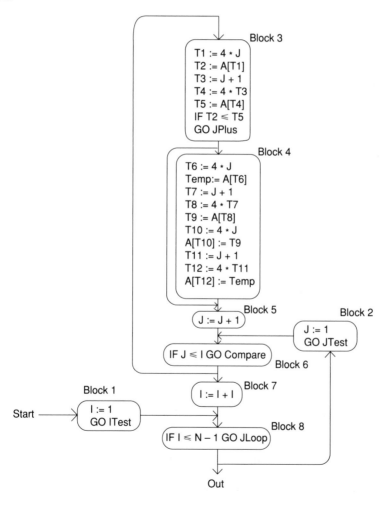

One of the best optimizations here would be an *algorithm optimization,* which would replace Bubblesort with a better algorithm such as Quicksort. We won't do this however.

There are algebraic optimizations here: T4 computes $4 * T3 = 4 * (J + 1) = 4 * J + 4$. Similarly, T8 computes $4 * T7 = 4 * (J + 1) = 4 * J + 4$ and $T12 = 4 * T11 = 4 * (J + 1) = 4 * J + 4$. Changing these:

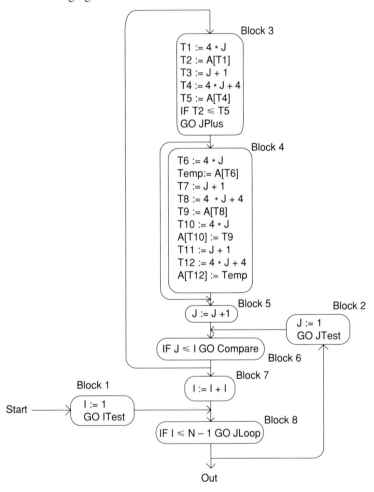

We look for some local optimizations which can be performed within the basic blocks.

There is *local common subexpression elimination* to be performed in our example. In Block 3, both T1 and T4 compute $4 * J$. In Block 4, T6, T8, T10, and T12 compute $4 * J$; both T7 and T11 compute $J + 1$; both T8 and T12 compute $4 * J + 4$.

We will replace the second occurrence of $4 * J$ in Block 3 by its value, T1, and the second, third and fourth occurrence in Block 4 by the computed value T6. T3, T7, and T11 go away:

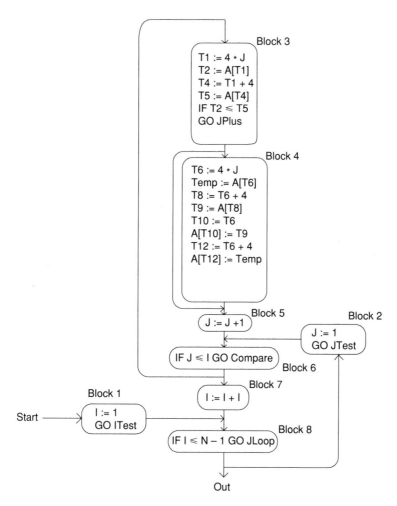

There is no opportunity for *local constant folding or elimination* unless *n* is known at compile time.

We move on to global and loop optimizations, presuming that data flow analysis has been performed (see Chapter 8, Exercise 2).

In Block 4, A[T6] which is A[4 ∗ J] is computed in Block 3. Control flow analysis tells us that we can't get to Block 4 without going through Block 3, and data flow analysis tells us that J doesn't change in between. Thus, we replace the first two statements in Block 4 by:

```
Temp := T2
```

Similarly, T10 is the same as T1, T8 is the same as T4, and T12 is the same as T4.

Block 4 becomes:

```
Temp := T1          A[T1] := T5
A[T1] := T5    →    A[T4] := T1
A[T4] := Temp
```

Looking at the revised program:

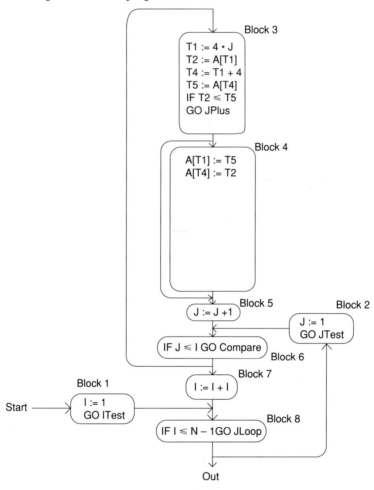

Next, we find the natural loops in order to perform induction-variable elimination. It is somewhat difficult to find the header of the inner loop because of the way the control flow graph is drawn, but Block 6 satisfies the definition from Chapter 7 (the reader is invited to check this). The loops are $\{6, 3, 4, 5\}$ and $\{2, 3, 4, 5, 6, 7, 8\}$.

For the loop, {Block 6, Block 3, Block 4, Block 5}, there are induction variables J (incremented by 1) and T1 and T4 (incremented by 4)

In Block 3:

```
T1 = 4 * J
T4 = 4 * J + 4
```

We can eliminate J, replacing the test on J with one on $T1$:

```
IF J ≤ I → IF T1 ≤ 4 * I
```

Note that J cannot be eliminated if it is to be used later in the program.

The new Block 6 becomes:

```
T14 := 4 * I
IF T1 ≤ T14 GO JLoop
```

In Block 2, we eliminate the initialization of *J* and replace it with a new Block 2:

```
T1 := 4
T4 := 8
```

Block 2 is functioning as a preheader here. We also need to replace the increment of *J* by an increment of T1 and T4. The new code is:

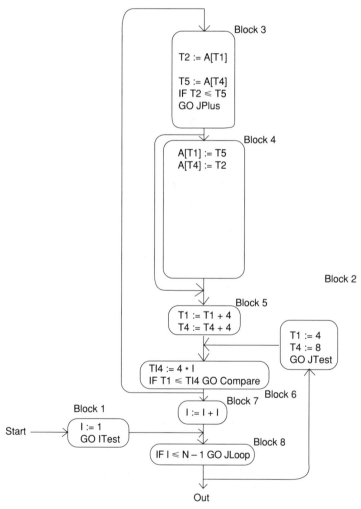

We now look for *loop invariants*.

```
T14 := 4 * I
```

is invariant in the inner loop, and we move it to Block 2:

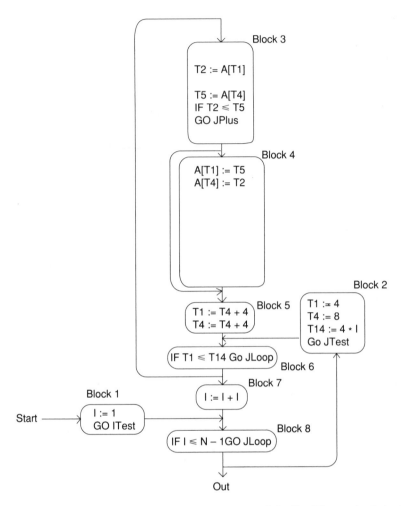

The final code is much improved over that shown originally. The reader is invited to search for more optimization to be performed here.

9.5   High-Level Optimization

Loveman (1977) describes the optimization phase as the "term given to the application of a set of rules for manipulating various representations of a program by exploiting local or global invariances within the program in order to improve the program relative to some measure."

In what follows, we assume a tree-structured representation and that the optimizations shown are really pattern-directed rearrangements of program text. As before, it is easier for humans to see this in source form or as quadruples.

The transformations are not applied in a random order; the successful application of one transformation suggests successor transformations. In fact, transformation ordering and information gathering is a major part of this method.

In addition, some transformations may not improve the program, but may lead to other transformations which do optimize. Similarly, some transformations may be machine-independent, but the reason for applying one may depend on the target machine.

9.5.1 Deduction of Program Invariances

The optimization process is viewed as deductions of program invariances such as "N has the value 4" or "this algorithm is executing on an 86-family machine" (see Exercise 12).

9.5.2 Program Measurement

The first step here (after parsing) is to determine whether or not optimization is in fact needed at all and, if so, where. The program might be remeasured after each transformation to see if it is worthwhile to continue.

9.5.3 Optimizations

The standard optimizations such as constant propagation, constant computation, common subexpression elimination, elimination of redundant code, etc. are tried. Primary interest, however, is on loops: removal of invariant code, strength reduction, case-splitting (described below), loop unrolling and fusion, and interaction between loops and conditionals.

Optimizations are viewed as containing seven parts: (1) the optimization name, (2) the pattern to be matched on the tree, (3) a pattern predicate which is true if the optimization preserves the semantics, (4) a win predicate if a transformation or a succeeding one improves the program, (5) pattern replacement rules, (6) predicate assertions which are true as a result of a transformation, (7) names of successor optimizations to try.

We illustrate all of this with an extended example.

9.5.4 High-Level Optimization: Example One

Consider the following program:

```
PROCEDURE Mult (in X: Matrix[L,M]; Y: Matrix[M,N];
                  out Z: Matrix[L,N])
  BEGIN {Mult}
    LOOP FOR I := 1 TO L DO
      BEGIN {ILoop}
        LOOP FOR J := 1 TO N DO
          BEGIN {JLoop}
            Z[I,J] := 0
            LOOP FOR K := 1 TO M DO
            BEGIN {KLoop}
              Z[I,J] := X[I,K] * Y[K,J] + Z[I,J]
            END {KLoop}
          END {JLoop}
      END {ILoop}
  END {Mult}
```

Suppose this procedure is called with *Mult(A,B,C)* and that the compiler ascertains that *A* is a 10 × 10 diagonal matrix, *B* is a 10 × 20 matrix and *N* is a 10 × 20 matrix. This information may be collected through programmer interaction or perhaps through reaching definitions and constant propagation and computation (see Exercise 13).

The expanded call is:

```
BEGIN {Mult}
  LOOP FOR I := 1 TO 10 DO
    BEGIN {ILoop}
      LOOP FOR J := 1 TO 20 DO
        BEGIN {JLoop}
          C[I,J] := 0
          LOOP FOR K := 1 TO 10 DO
          BEGIN {KLoop}
            C[I,J] := A[I,K] * B[K,J] + C[I,J]
          END {KLoop}
        END {JLoop}
    END {ILoop}
END {Mult}
```

We can perform an optimization called *case-splitting* by replacing

```
A[I,K]
```

by

```
IF I ≠ K THEN 0
ELSE A[I,K]
```

in the innermost loop:

```
BEGIN {Mult}
  LOOP FOR I := 1 TO 10 DO
    BEGIN {ILoop}
      LOOP FOR J := 1 TO 20 DO
        BEGIN {JLoop}
          C[I,J] := 0
          LOOP FOR K := 1 TO 10 DO
          BEGIN {KLoop}
            IF I ≠ K THEN
              C[I,J] := 0 * B[K,J] + C[I,J]
            ELSE
              C[I,J] := A[I,K] * B[K,J] + C[I,J]
          END {KLoop}
        END {JLoop}
    END {ILoop}
END {Mult}
```

The THEN clause, after constant computation, is C[I,J] := C[I,J], which may be removed. The ELSE clause becomes a THEN clause by changing the test to *IF I = K*. In the (new) THEN clause, all references to K are replaced by I

```
BEGIN {Mult}
  LOOP FOR I := 1 TO 10 DO
    BEGIN {ILoop}
      LOOP FOR J := 1 TO 20 DO
        BEGIN {JLoop}
          C[I,J] := 0
          LOOP FOR K := 1 TO 10 DO
            BEGIN {KLoop}
              IF I = K THEN
              C[I,J] := A[I,I] * B[I,J] + C[I,J]
            END {KLoop}
        END {JLoop}
    END {ILoop}
END {Mult}
```

I and J are basic induction variables, and we can simplify further by calculating when I = K. In general, for

```
LOOP FOR I := I_initial TO I_final DO
...
  LOOP FOR K := K_initial TO K_final
    IF I = K THEN...
  ENDLOOP K
ENDLOOP I
```

the values of I and K intersect if $I_{initial} \leq K_{final}$ and $K_{initial} \leq I_{final}$.
  The value of I in the innermost loop is within the intersection if

$$\text{Max}(K_{initial}, I_{initial}) \leq I$$

and

$$I \leq \text{Min}(K_{final}, I_{final})$$

Using this transformation, the program now becomes

```
BEGIN {Mult}
  LOOP FOR I := 1 TO 10 DO
    BEGIN {ILoop}
      LOOP FOR J := 1 TO 20 DO
        BEGIN {JLoop}
          C[I,J] := 0
          IF 1 ≤ 10 AND 1 ≤ 10 AND Max(1,1) ≤ I
            AND I ≤ Min(10,10) THEN
              C[I,J] := A[I,I] * B[I,J] + C[I,J]
        END {JLoop}
    END {ILoop}
END {Mult}
```

The statements in the IF statement can be computed by the compiler using constant computation yielding:

```
BEGIN {Mult}
  LOOP FOR I := 1 TO 10 DO
    BEGIN {I Loop}
      LOOP FOR J := 1 TO 20 DO
        BEGIN {J Loop}
          C[I,J] := 0
          C[I,J] := A[I,I] * B[I,J] + C[I,J]
        END {JLoop}
    END {ILoop}
END {Mult}
```

We can propagate the constant C[I,J] = 0 and eliminate the dead code:

```
BEGIN {Mult}
  LOOP FOR I := 1 TO 10 DO
    BEGIN {ILoop}
      LOOP FOR J := 1 TO 20 DO
        BEGIN {JLoop}
          C[I,J] := A[I,I] * B[I,J]
        END {JLoop}
    END {ILoop}
END {Mult}
```

The final version is much simpler than the original. The next example computes a matrix expression.

9.5.5   High-Level Optimization: Example Two

Consider procedures *Plus*

```
PROCEDURE Plus(in X : Matrix[L,M], Y: Matrix[L,M];
                        out Z: Matrix{L,M} )
  BEGIN {Plus}
    LOOP FOR I := 1 TO L DO
      BEGIN {I Loop}
      LOOP FOR J := 1 TO M DO
        BEGIN {J Loop}
          Z[I,J] := X[I,J] + Y[I,J]
        END {J Loop}
      END {ILoop}
  END {Plus}
```

and *Assign*

```
PROCEDURE Assign(in X : Matrix[L,M]; out Z:
                                            Matrix{L,M})
  BEGIN {Assign}
    LOOP FOR I := 1 TO L DO
      BEGIN {ILoop}
```

```
    LOOP FOR J := 1 TO M DO
      BEGIN {JLoop}
        Z[I,J] := X[I,J]
      END {JLoop}
    END {ILoop}
  END {Assign}
```

Suppose *A*, *B*, *C*, and *D* are 10×10 matrices, and we want to compute the matrix expression

```
D := (A * B) + C
```

We do this by the sequence of matrix calls:

```
Mult(A, B, T1)
Plus(T1, C, T2)
Assign(T2, D)
```

The expanded program is:

```
BEGIN {Mult}
  LOOP FOR I := 1 TO 10 DO
    BEGIN {ILoop}
      LOOP FOR J := 1 TO 10 DO
        BEGIN {JLoop}
          T1[I,J] := 0
          LOOP FOR K := 1 TO 10 DO
            BEGIN {KLoop}
              T1[I,J] := A[I,K] * B[K,J] + T1[I,J]
            END {KLoop}
        END {JLoop}
    END {ILoop}
END {Mult}
BEGIN {Plus}
  LOOP FOR I := 1 TO 10 DO
    BEGIN {ILoop}
      LOOP FOR J := 1 TO 10 DO
        BEGIN {JLoop}
          T2[I,J] := T1[I,J] + C[I,J]
        END {JLoop}
    END {ILoop}
END {Plus}
BEGIN {Assign}
  LOOP FOR I := 1 TO 10 DO
    BEGIN {ILoop}
      LOOP FOR J := 1 TO 10 DO
        BEGIN {JLoop}
          D[I,J] := T2[I,J]
        END {JLoop}
    END {ILoop}
END {Assign}
```

The three outer loops may be fused since the index sets are the same and there are no data dependencies.

```
BEGIN {A * B + C}
  LOOP FOR I := 1 TO 10 DO
    BEGIN {ILoop}
      LOOP FOR J := 1 TO 10 DO
        BEGIN {JLoop}
          T1[I,J] := 0
          LOOP FOR K := 1 TO 10 DO
            BEGIN {KLoop}
              T1[I,J] := A[I,K] * B[K,J] + T1[I,J]
            END {KLoop}
              T2[I,J] := T1[I,J] + C[I,J]
              D[I,J] := T2[I,J]
        END {JLoop}
    END {ILoop}
END {A * B + C}
```

Each instance of *T1[I,J]* is dead after the ith and jth iteration of the two outer loops, that is *T1* and *T2* are really scalars. We perform a *subsumption*, that is, we replace a variable which is used once by its definition, and initialize *T1* to *C[I,J]*:

```
BEGIN {A * B + C}
  LOOP FOR I := 1 TO 10 DO
    BEGIN {Loop}
      LOOP FOR J := 1 TO 10 DO
        BEGIN {JLoop}
          T1[I,J] := C[I,J]
          LOOP FOR K := 1 TO 10 DO
            BEGIN {KLoop}
              T1[I,J] := A[I,K] * B[K,J] + T1
            END {KLoop}
              D[I,J] := T1
        END {JLoop}
    END {ILoop}
END {A * B + C}
```

We could eliminate *T1* entirely, but then we would have to substitute array references which is costly.

In the next section, we discuss how these examples might be implemented using pattern matching.

9.5.6 Implementation

We can create a table of optimizations indexed by name consisting of the seven parts described in Section 9.5.2. Each entry might be of the form

```
(1) Name:  (2) in pattern (3) where pattern predicate
           (4) when win predicate
```

(5) **then** pattern$_1$ → replacement$_1$

   ...

   pattern$_n$ → replacement$_n$

(6) **assert** predicate$_1$, predicate$_2$...
                         predicate$_k$

(7) **nowtry** Name$_1$, Name$_2$, ...Name$_m$

Not all optimizations will have all seven parts. The optimization *IsAConstant* would be:

(1) **IsAConstant:** (2) **in** "x := y" (3) **where** "y is a constant"

          (6) **assert** constant(x), value(x) = value(y)

          (7) **nowtry** DeadVariableElimination, PropagateConstant

The optimization *PropagateConstant* would be:

(1) **PropagateConstant:** (2) **in** "x" (3) **where**
              constant(x)

           (5) **then** replace x with value(x)

           (7) **nowtry** ConstantComputation, IsAConstant

The optimization *ConstantComputation* is:

(1) **ConstantComputation:** (2) **in** "x op y" (3) **where**
                IsAConstant(x) AND IsAConstant(y)

             (5) **then** replace x op y with value(x) op value(y)

             (7) nowtry ConstantComputation, IsAConstant

The optimization *DeadVariable* is:

(1) **DeadVariableElimination:** (2) **in** "x :=y" (3) **where**
                   dead(x)

              (5) **then** replace x := y with null

The above transformations had no win predicates since they always result in program improvement. Exercise 14 asks the reader to create more of these table entries.

9.6 Optimization Statistics

This chapter has discussed a large number of optimizations, most of which are found on the control flow graph. The reader may be wondering what the improvements really are. Is it worth the time and effort at compile time—not to mention at compiler creation time—to perform such aggressive optimizations?

The answer is—it depends. Statistics have shown that there is a 5–25% improvement in running time for the loop optimizations:

- Code motion of loop invariant statements
- Induction variable elimination

There is a 1–5% improvement for:

- Global common subexpression elimination
- Dead variable detection
- Use of algebraic laws
- Constant propagation

Interestingly, the topic of the next chapter, register allocation, has been shown to improve code more than the optimizations above. Because good register allocation does improve code, it is often discussed in chapters on optimization.

The optimizations performed after code generation, peephole optimization, also have a high payoff. We discuss these in Chapter 10.

9.7   Interprocedural Optimization

Procedure calls may be approached in two ways. The first is to assume the worst case for the call, and the second is to actually perform the data flow analyses throughout the procedure.

For the first approach, default assumptions include assuming no definitions are killed, expressions are no longer available, etc.

Approach two requires careful following of *aliases*. An alias is another name for a location. Reference parameters are aliases for the actual arguments. Once aliases are identified, the analysis is similar to intraprocedural analysis.

9.8   Summary

This chapter has used the results of the last two chapters to improve programs so that the ultimate code executes faster. In some cases, this also performs a space improvement; in some cases the improvement in time produces code which consumes more space.

We divide these improvements into three categories: local, loop and global. The divisions are somewhat arbitrary in that loop optimizations may be classified as either local or global. Loop optimizations, in general, improve code more that other optimizations.

There are two more improvements, often categorized as optimizations because they improve program performance greatly: good register allocation and peephole optimization (see Chapter 10).

9.9   Related Reading

Allen, F. E. and J. Cocke. 1971. A Catalogue of Optimizing Transformations, in R. Rustin (ed), *Design and Optimization of Compilers*, 1–31.

Allen, F. E., J. Cocke, and K. Kennedy. 1979. Reduction of Operator Strength, in S. Muchnick and N. Jones (eds.) *Program Flow Analysis: Theory and Applications*, Englewood Cliffs, NJ: Prentice-Hall, 79–101.

Allen, F., B. Rosen, and K. Zadeck. 1990. Optimization in Compilers, ACM Press/Addison-Wesley.

Callahan, D., K. Cooper, K. Kennedy, and L. Torczon. 1986. *Interprocedural Constant Propagation*, in Proceedings of the ACM SIGPLAN Symposium on Compiler Construction, 20–24.

Cytron, R., A. Lowry, and K. Zadeck. 1986. *Code Motion of Control Structures in High-Level Languages*, 70–85.

Davidson, J. W. and C. W. Fraser. 1982. *Elimination of Redundant Object Code*, in POPL Conference Proceedings, 128–32.

Dhamdere, D. M. 1991. Practical Adaptation of the Global Optimization Algorithm of Morel and Renvoise, *ACM Transactions on Programming Languages and Systems*, 13(2):292–294.

Knuth, D. E. 1971. An Empirical Study of FORTRAN Programs, *Software Practice and Experience*, 1(12):105–134.

Kuck, D., R. Kuhn, D. Padua, B. Leasure, and M. Wolfe. 1981. *Dependence Graphs and Compiler Optimizations*, POPL Conference Proceedings, 207–218.

Loveman, D. 1977. Program Improvement by Source-to-Source Transformation, *Journal of the ACM*, 24(1).
  Presents a high-level view of the optimization process as well as an extensive "catalogue" of optimizations.

Massalin, H. 1987. *Superoptimizer: A Look at the Smallest Program*, ASPLOS II, 122–126.

Wegman, M. and F. Zadeck. 1991. Constant Propagation with Conditional Branches, *ACM Transactions on Programming Languages and Systems*, 13(2):181–210.

Wulf et al. 1975. *The Design of an Optimizing Compiler*, New York: Elsevier North-Holland.

EXERCISES

1. Perform a strength reduction on:
   (a) `A := 8 * I`
   (b) `A := I`^{2}

2. Assuming quadruple intermediate representation, write an algorithm to perform
   (a) Constant folding as in Example 4
   (b) Constant folding in Example 5

3. What changes need to be made to perform constant folding if the intermediate representation is an abstract syntax tree?

4. What other optimizations might be included in a general constant folding test?

5. Why is the statement $X := Y + Z$ in Example 7 not loop-invariant?

6. Eliminate variable i in Example 12 by replacing the FOR loop with a WHILE loop, making all the appropriate changes.

7. Name some other strength reductions.

8. Can the following loops be fused?

```
LOOP I := 1 to 100
   A(I) := 0
ENDLOOP
LOOP I := 1 to 100
   A(I) = A(I) + Y
ENDLOOP
```

9. Write an algorithm to find and implement each of the following optimizations. Presume control flow analysis and data flow analysis have been performed and that there are procedures to call to find loop invariants and induction variables.
   (a) Loop unrolling
   (b) Loop fusion
   (c) Unswitching

10. For the program in Section 9.4,
    (a) Find the dominators.
    (b) Perform a data flow analysis.
    (c) Show that the two loops described are natural loops.
    (d) Explain what information is needed (from (b) and (c)) in order to perform each of the optimizations discussed in Section 9.4.

    or

    (e) For each of the optimizations discussed, write an algorithm outline (using dominators, reaching definitions, live variable analysis, etc.) to find the optimization.

11. Following the outline in Section 9.4, create the basic blocks and the control flow graph, perform data flow analyses and optimize the following algorithm which performs an *exchange* sort:

```
LOOP FOR I := 1 TO N - 1
   Min := List_i
   Place := i
   LOOP FOR J := i + 1 TO N
      IF List_j < Min THEN
         Place := J
         Min := List_j
      ENDIF
   ENDLOOP J
   Temp := List_i
   List_i := List_Place
   List_Place := Temp
ENDLOOP
```

12. Name other program invariances as discussed in Section 9.5.1.

13. Using data flow analysis, show how a compiler might discover that a matrix is a diagonal matrix.

14. Create table entries for the following using the models in Section 9.5.6:
    (a) algebraic simplifications such as multiplying by one and adding zero
    (b) loop collapsing
    (c) conditional pruning
    (d) conditional reordering
    (e) goto chasing
    (f) elimination of array temporaries
    (g) hoisting of loop-invariants
    (h) induction-variable elimination
    (i) replacement of loop conditional with a count up to 0
    (j) movement of While test to loop end
    (k) strip mining
    (l) loop unrolling

10

Code Generation
Techniques

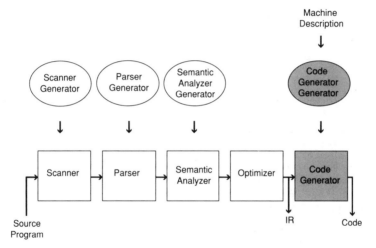

10.0   Introduction

The code generation phase translates the intermediate representation into "code". In this chapter, the final code will be assembly language. A production quality compiler would, most likely, produce object code, and this is discussed in Chapter 11.

Three phases can be identified as part of the code generation phase: (1) preparation for code generation, (2) code selection and (3) "peephole" optimization.

True code generator generators are still evolving, although much research has been devoted to this topic. Retargetable code generators or table-driven code generators are becoming more common. They enable a code generator to be created for a new machine with relative ease by separating the code generation algorithm (the driver) from the machine description. This is similar to the front-end generators which we saw in earlier chapters.

The preparation for code generation phase decides how to allocate registers; code selection translates the intermediate representation to assembly language; peephole optimization peeps at small sections of the resulting code to see if improvements can be made. We will discuss each of these in the sections that follow.

10.1   Register Allocation

To prepare for code generation, the compiler decides where values of variables and expressions will reside during execution. The preferred location is a register since instructions execute faster when the data referred to in operands reside in registers. Ultimate storage is often a memory location, and due to the scarcity of registers, even intermediate results may need to be assigned memory locations also.

Memory allocation techniques are discussed in Chapter 11; in this chapter, we will address the issue of register allocation.

10.1.1   Register Allocation vs. Assignment

The term *register allocation* is used for two tasks: (1) *register allocation* itself which decides which program values shall reside in registers and (2) *register assignment* which picks the specific register in which these values will reside.

Some compilers make a tentative allocation, then try an assignment, and if necessary reallocate.

10.1.2   Register Allocation Schemes

A good code generator will generate code that minimizes accesses to main memory; it will try to keep as much currently active data (values of variables and expressions) in registers as possible.

There are two general approaches to register allocation. The first divides the registers to be allocated into two classes. The first class is those globally allocated: those to be allocated for the whole program or for a whole subprogram or perhaps a loop, and the second class is those used for temporary values and computations within a straight-line (no branches from IF's or loops) sequence of code.

The second method is to do *all* allocation on a global basis, without dividing the registers into two classes.

Simple global register allocation allocates registers for variables in inner loops first since that is generally where a program spends a lot of its time. Of course, this same register should be used for the variable if it also appears in an outer loop. After registers have been allocated globally, at least one (and often more) register is kept free for holding temporary results.

10.1.3   Register Allocation by Usage Counts

A slightly more sophisticated method for global register allocation is called *usage counts*. (This is a heuristic. A heuristic method is one that usually, but not always, makes things better.) In this method, registers are allocated first to the variables that are used the most.

EXAMPLE 1   Allocation using usage counts

Consider the following loop:

```
LOOP X := 2 * E
     Z := Y + X + 1
     IF some condition THEN
     Y := Z + Y
```

```
         D := Y - 1
     ELSE Z := X - Y
       D := 2
     ENDIF
     X := Z + D
   ENDLOOP
```

Here, there are four references to *X* and *Z*, five references to *Y*, three reference to *D* and one to *E*. Thus, if there are three registers, a reasonable approach would be to allocate *X* and *Z* to two of them, saving the third for local computations. The resulting code would be (something like):

```
     Load X,R1
     Load Z,R2
LOOP Load E, R3
     Mult #2,R3
     Store R3,X
     Copy R1,R3
     Add Y,R3
     Add #1,R3
     Store R3,Z
     IF some condition THEN
       Copy R2,R3
       Add Y,R3
       Store R3,Y
       Load Y,R3
       Sub #1,R3
       Store R3,D
     ELSE Copy R1,R3
       Sub Y,R3
       Store R3,Z
       Load #2,R3
       Store R3,D
     ENDIF
       Copy R2,R3
       Add D,R3
       Store R3,X
ENDLOOP
```

Of course, there would be compare and branch instructions for the IF's and LOOPS.

A more complex method for register allocation is allocation by graph coloring.

10.1.4   Register Allocation and Assignment by Graph Coloring

Register allocation by coloring uses def-use chains from data flow analysis to find what variables and expressions can share registers. A def-use chain consists of an assignment to a variable or a computation of the value of an expression and all its uses. Two program quantities cannot share the same registers if their def-use chains overlap. Such program quantities are said to share overlapping *lifetimes*.

If *n* is the number of available registers, and *ColorGraph(n)* is a procedure which tries to color the graph using *n* colors, the algorithm is:

Algorithm
Register Allocation by Coloring
```
For each program quantity to be allocated to a register DO
  Create a node
Draw an arc between nodes whose lifetimes overlap
ColorGraph(n)
```

If the graph can be colored with *n* colors, then the allocation is possible, and these *n* registers can now be assigned. The graph is called an *interference graph*.

Graph coloring is an NP-complete problem when *n* is greater than two, meaning no polynomial algorithm is known for the worst case. Most often, a worst case is not encountered, however, and the usual method is to use a greedy algorithm (see Exercise 9). Exercise 10 asks the reader to draw the interference graph for the program of Example 1.

10.1.5   Register Assignment and Reassignment

Register allocation assigns a priority to which values are to be kept in registers. The other side of this problem is which registers to use for these values. Sometimes the machine requires that a certain register be used for certain operations, as in the 86-family where registers AX and DX are used in multiply and divide instructions.

Registers are allocated and then freed when the value assigned is no longer needed. On the other hand, when we run out of registers at a certain point in a program, we may need to remove a value that is in a register to use that register for a value that is more important.

Removing a value from a register is called a register *spill*. In general, if any registers contain small constants, these registers would be spilled first (since most machines have *immediate* instructions which calculate the values of constants). If a value in a register is the same as its stored value, then this is a reasonable value to remove because no *store* instruction needs to be generated. Variables and expressions which will not be referenced again might be removed next. Data flow analysis techniques can find these.

A heuristic often used is Belady's algorithm, which is a variant of an operating system algorithm used to find free space in paging systems.

Algorithm
Belady's Algorithm Adapted for Register Allocation
```
IF the required value is already in an acceptable place THEN
  leave it there
ELSE IF there is an acceptable empty register THEN
  choose it
ELSE use that acceptable register whose value will not be
  used for the longest time and move this value to main memory
```

Clearly, the majority of the work done by this algorithm is in the second ELSE.

EXAMPLE 2 Using Belady's algorithm

Suppose a program refers to the variables *u, v, w,* and *x* as follows:

```
u v w x v u x v x w
```

There is a reference to *u* then a reference to *v*, then a reference to *w*, etc.

Suppose further that we have 3 registers to use, R1, R2, and R3. The variable *u* will be assigned to R1, *v* to R2, *w* to R3, and then we have a problem with the reference to *x*. Scanning the list, we see that *w* is not used for the longest time; there are references to *u* and *v* before a reference to *w*. Thus, *w* gets spilled from register 3 and *x* is loaded into register 3.

The assignments are as follows:

Variable Reference	R1	R2	R3
u	u		
v		v	
w			w
x			x
v		v	
u	u		
x			x
v		v	
x			x
w	(can go into any register)		

Another commonly used heuristic (also used in paging systems) is to store the variable that has not been used for the longest time; thus, the algorithm examines the past references instead of the future uses (see Exercise 1).

10.1.6 Register Management

There is much bookkeeping to keep track of how registers are used at various program points. Often, one needs to keep track of current and future register use. The following is useful information for registers which are not free:

1. Description of contents
2. Future uses (usage count)
3. Distance to next use
4. Copy in memory?
5. Copy in another register?
6. Cost of recomputing contents
7. Most recent use
8. Past uses

In summary, register allocation and management can be simple or complex. The same is true of code generation itself.

10.2 Code Generation

Selecting code and allocating registers is a chicken and egg problem, as the registers that are used influence the code and vice versa. For now, however, we will assume that register allocation has already taken place.

Good code generation produces code that executes fast or takes up less space. Such code generation is very difficult. But it is easy to write a naive code generator. One merely writes an algorithm to translate the intermediate code, fetching and storing as needed. Even register allocation is not necessary.

Since the algorithm is so simple, we leave it to the exercises and illustrate it with an example.

EXAMPLE 3   Quick 'n dirty code generation

Consider the following abstract syntax tree for the two assignment statements

```
X1 := A + BB * 12 ;
X2 := A/2 + BB * 12 ;
```

from earlier chapters:

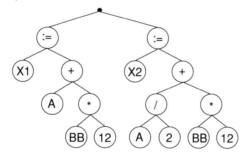

Using a depth-first tree walk, the following code can be easily produced:

```
Load    BB,R1
Mult    #12,R1
Store   R1,Temp1
Load    A,R1
Add     Temp1,R1
Store   R1,Temp2
Load    Temp2,R1
Store   R1,X1
Load    A,R1
Div     R1,#2
Store   R1,Temp3
Load    BB,R1
```

```
Mult    #12,R1
Store   T4,R1
Load    T3,R1
Add     T4,R1
Store   T5,R1
Load    T5,R1
Store   R1,X1
```

The code in Example 3 contains numerous inefficiencies (see Exercise 2). A good code generator would not have produced these inefficiencies, and/or a peephole optimizer would find them and eliminate them.

10.3 Instruction Selection from Intermediate Representations

There are numerous intermediate representations (IR), that is, there are numerous possibilities for the input to the code generator. This, of course, influences the code generation algorithms. In this chapter, we will presume that the IR is an abstract syntax tree.

The symbol table is used to generate directives. Thus if variable *A* is entered in the symbol table as having a class of integer, then the directive that allocates space for an integer is generated. Example 4 shows directives for integers for a number of machines.

EXAMPLE 4 Directives for a symbol table entry with class integer and character string *A*

```
On the Vax:          A:  .LONG
On the 86-family:    A   DW  ?
On the M68000:       A   DS.L
```

The VAX directive and the M68000 allocate 32 bits in memory for the variable *A*. The 86-family directives allocate 16 bits in memory for the variable *A*. None of these directives assigns an initial value (although it is possible to do so).

It is often convenient to change the code for conditionals and loops in intermediate representations (such as abstract syntax trees) to the lower level form with jumps (GOTO's), as seen in representations such as three-address code. This is called *code lowering*.

It is hard to build a *good* code generator. Essentially, it is a large case analysis. We show code for some common constructs.

10.3.1 Standard Code Generation Strategies

A code generator can be written to recognize standard templates. In the following, we use an assembly language notation which assumes that the first operand is the *source* and the second operand is the *destination*.

(1) Assignment Statements

A tree pattern of the form

generates a Move (Copy) instruction:

```
MOVE APlace,T
```

or

```
MOVE APlace,Reg
MOVE Reg,T
```

where *APlace* represents the register or memory location assigned to *A*.

(2) Arithmetic Operations

Suppose *op* represents an arithmetic operation and consider an abstract syntax tree for the statement $T := A\ op\ B$:

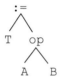

One possible code sequence is:

```
MOVE    APlace,Reg
OP      BPlace,Reg
MOVE    Reg,T
```

Of course, some machines require special registers be used for some operations such as multiplication and division.

Example 5 shows code for the instruction $T := A - B$

EXAMPLE 5   Code for $T := A - B$

An abstract syntax tree is:

Following the template above yields:

```
MOVE      APlace,Reg
SUBTRACT  BPlace,Reg
MOVE      Reg,T
```

Here the SUBTRACT instruction subtracts the first operand from the second.

(3) **IF Statements**

IF statements can be represented by an abstract syntax tree such as:

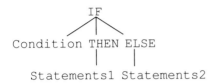

```
              IF
            ╱  │  ╲
Condition THEN ELSE
             │    │
        Statements1 Statements2
```

A typical code sequence is

```
            (Code for condition)
            BRANCHIFFALSE Label1
            (Code for Statements1)
            BRANCH Label2
Label1: (Code for Statements2)
Label2:
```

Example 6 illustrates this for the statement:

```
IF  A < B THEN Max := B ELSE Max := A
```

EXAMPLE 6   IF A < B THEN Max := B ELSE Max := A

The abstract syntax tree is:

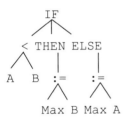

```
       IF
     ╱ │ ╲
   < THEN ELSE
  ╱╲  │    │
 A  B :=    :=
     ╱╲   ╱╲
   Max B Max A
```

Following the model above, the code would be:

```
COMPARE     APlace,BPlace    ; (Code for comparison)
BGEQ        Label1           ; NOT <
MOVE        BPlace,Max       ; (Code for Statements1)
BRANCH      Label2
Label1:     MOVE APlace,Max  ; (Code for Statements2)
Label2:
```

---

(4) **Loops**

In some sense, loops are just conditionals whose code is repeated. Consider the loop:

```
LOOP While condition DO
      Statements
ENDLOOP
```

An abstract syntax tree is:

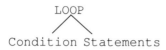

```
        LOOP
       /    \
Condition  Statements
```

A reasonable code sequence might be:

```
Label1:  (Code for NOT condition)
         BRANCHIFTRUE  Label2
         (Code for Statements)
         BRANCH  Label1
Label2:
```

Example 7 shows such a loop.

EXAMPLE 7   Code for *WHILE A < B DO X := 3*

The abstract syntax tree is:

```
    WHILE
    /   \
   <    :=
  / \  / \
 A  B X   3
```

A possible code sequence is:

```
Label1:  COMPARE    A, B
         BRANCHGE   Label2
         MOVE       #3, X
         GOTO       Label1
Label2:
```

Here, the NOT has been incorporated into the conditional branch, BRANCHGE, pseudocode for "Branch on Greater Than or Equal To".

(5) Array References

Most machines today have instructions that perform indexing. Consider the statement:

```
A := B[I]
```

An abstract syntax tree might be:

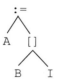

```
     :=
    /  \
   A   []
       / \
      B   I
```

If the machine has indirect addressing, one code sequence is:

```
MOVEADDRESS    B,Reg1
MOVE           I,Reg2
MOVE           Reg2(Reg1),A
```

Here, we have produced code for a machine that has indirect addressing. If Reg1 contains an address, *Addr1*, and Reg2 contains a value, *Val1*, then the notation *Reg2(Reg1)* refers to *Addr1 + Val1*. Many machines have such addressing modes.

Exercise 8 explores other code generation templates.

10.4   An Efficient Register Allocator and Code Generator for Expressions

The following algorithm writes, on each tree node of an expression tree, the number of registers needed to compute the node. It assumes a computer model that requires one of the operands to be in a register. Thus left-most leaves are assigned a 1, and right-most leaves are assigned a 0 (it could be reversed). Parent nodes are assigned the maximum of the values of both children. If the values are equal, one more register is needed to store the result, so the parent node is assigned the (equal) value plus one.

Algorithm
Label(ExpressionNode)
```
1. Node is a left-most leaf: Label# = 1
2. Node is a right-most leaf: Label# = 0
3. (Otherwise) Label(Left(Node))
        Label(Right(Node))
        Label#(Node) = Max(Left Label#,Right Label#)
        or Left Label# + 1 if Left Label# = Right Label#
```

The algorithm is called with Label(Root)

Example 8 illustrates the labeling algorithm by computing the number of registers needed to compute $(A * B) + (C + D) * (E + F)$.

EXAMPLE 8   Labeling a tree for the expression $(A * B) + (C + D) * (E + F)$

Following the algorithm above, the labeled abstract tree is:

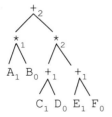

Thus, two registers are needed (and are sufficient) to compute this expression.

Using a tree labeled as above, we can write a code generation algorithm.

Algorithm

GenerateCode(*Node*)

```
CASE Node
Is a leaf labeled 1, and a left leaf:
  (a) R := GetReg
  (b) Generate "LOAD Node, R"
Is labeled with a # greater than available registers:
  (a) Generate code for right child
  (b) Store result in a Temp
  (c) Generate code for left child
  (e) Apply Node's operator to (a) and (c)
Has a right child that is a leaf:
  (a) Evaluate left child
  (b) Apply Node's operator to left child result and
      leaf.
(Otherwise)
  (a) Apply code generation to Node with larger
      label. If they are the same, then it doesn't
      matter. Leave the result in register.
  (b) Apply code generation to remaining child.
  (c) Apply Node's operation to registers holding the
      two results.
```

Example 9 generates code for the expression of Example 7.

EXAMPLE 9   Generating code for (A * B) + (C + D) * (E + F)

Using the labeled tree in Example 8 and the code generation algo-rithm yields:

```
LOAD     C, Reg1
ADD      D, Reg1
LOAD     E, Reg2
ADD      F, Reg2
MULT     Reg1, Reg2
LOAD     A, Reg1
MULT     B, Reg1
ADD      Reg2, Reg1
```

Exercise 3 explores how to change this in order to generate code for other con-structs such as assignment statements, conditionals and loops.

10.5   Code Generation from DAGs

The optimal code generation algorithm is an NP-complete problem. Directed acyclic graphs allow a code Generation heuristic:

> Put out code for each node immediately after code for its children has
> been emitted as far as possible because then the results are more apt to
> still be available, say in a register.

To prepare the list of DAG nodes to compute (that is, the list for which code is to be emitted), start at the root of the right-most subtree. Put this node on the list, L, and continue by adding a left-most node to the list after all its parents are already on the list. Then generate code for the nodes in L by starting at the end of L and proceeding to the beginning.

EXAMPLE 10   Generating code from a DAG

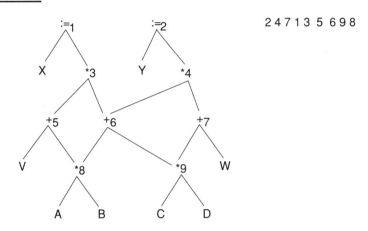

2 4 7 1 3 5 6 9 8

Thus, we would put out code for node 8 first, then node 9, etc.

Another way to put out good code from DAG's is to break the DAG up into trees and to use a code generation algorithm which is optimal on trees. (Of course, it takes time to break up the DAG.)

EXAMPLE 11   Breaking DAGs into trees

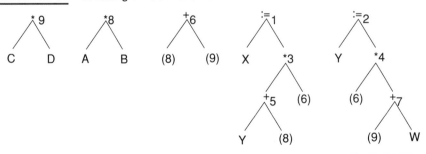

10.6   **Retargetable Code Generation**

Retargetable code generation is a step toward automatic code generation. The code generator is designed so that it can be changed to produce code for a new machine. These may be categorized (Ganapathi et al., 1982) as (1) interpretive code generators, (2) pattern matching code generators and (3) table-driven code generators. In all of these, an attempt is made to separate the code generation algorithm from the machine code itself. This fits our model of a driver and the information on which the driver operates with the code generation algorithm analogous to the driver.

10.6.1   Interpretive Code Generators

Interpretive code generators are either hand-written translators (some P-code trans-lators) or schema-driven (U-code translators) translators which implement a map-ping between virtual machine instructions and real machine instructions. Such retar-getable code generators separate the code generation algorithm from the target language somewhat, but are often too closely tied to a specific language or a specific machine.

It is also difficult to incorporate context-dependent information such as differenti-ating between Booleans and assignment statements. For example, the Boolean expression $B < C$ in

```
A := B < C
```

may need to be stored (for a future use) while in

```
IF B < C THEN ...
```

the Boolean expression does not need to be saved; code to set the machines's condi-tion codes is emitted. Interpretive code generators find such context-dependent infor-mation difficult to identify.

10.6.2   Pattern Matching Code Generators

Although all code generation is, to some extent, pattern matching, the first pattern matching code generators separated the machine code descriptions from the code generation algorithm and avoided interpretation by creating a single tree structure called a pattern tree to encode all potential instructions. The code generation algo-rithm then walked the IR tree, trying to find a match in the pattern tree.

These code generators tend to be slow. Special rules which convert the tree so that $1 + a$ is treated the same as $a + 1$ aid the matching process, but also slow it down.

10.6.3   Table-Driven Code Generation

Table-driven methods attempt to automate the pattern matching process. They tend to be more flexible and easier to finely tune. Many of these approaches separate the register allocation from the instruction selection.

Method of Cattell

One method, developed by Cattell (1980), creates a table of ordered pairs (*IR node, machine code to be produced*). These ordered pairs are ordered so that a more effi-cient special case is tried first. For example, the patterns below might be a subset of the patterns which match an IR node whose operator is "+". The IR pattern:

would produce the code

```
INC X
```

while the IR pattern

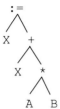

would produce the code:

```
(Code for *)
ADD TimesPlace,Reg
```

if the code for * left its result in *TimesPlace*. The ordered pairs that produce the code for * are also stored in the table.

Because of the subtargeting process, this method has been criticized as not separating the code from the code generation algorithm.

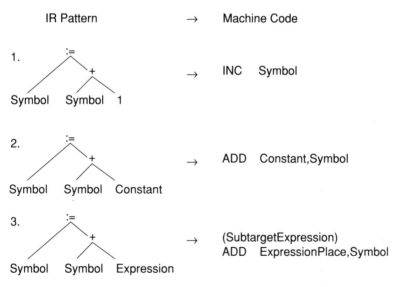

Here, *SubtargetExpression* puts out code for Expression, leaving the result in *ExpressionPlace*.

Method of Ganapathi

The method of Ganapathi is an extension of a method developed by Glanville (1977) and Graham (1978, 1980) in the late 1970's. Basically, the method is to parse the IR, producing code in the same sense that the source program is parsed producing IR.

This means that the IR itself must be described by using a grammar. For example, the production

```
Byte → + Byte Byte
```

describes an abstract syntax tree node which says that a byte operation can be the operator "+" and two byte operands. Looking at this in another way, we can say that the sum of two byte operands is itself a byte.

Ganapathi adds synthesized attributes to these productions:

```
Byte ↑ x → + Byte ↑ x Byte ↑ y
```

where the up-arrows serve as visual reminders that the attributes are synthesized. Here, attributes x and y might indicate that the storage location for the first operand, x, is to be used for the sum. Predicates may also be used:

```
Byte ↑ x → + Byte ↑ x Byte ↑ y          IsOne (↓ y)
```

The down-arrow here indicates that the ingoing argument for y is to be used. This predicate states that a match takes place only if the second operand on the abstract syntax tree is the constant "1". (There will be other productions for the other cases.)

Code is emitted by adding *actions*:

```
Byte ↑ x → + Byte ↑ x Byte ↑ y IsOne (↓ y) EMIT
                                  (↓ "INCB" ↓X)
```

Here, the action emits the code *INCB XPlace*, where the information about XPlace is contained in the attribute X.

To find the case when the first operand is one:

```
Byte ↑ x → + Byte ↑ x Byte ↑ y IsOne (↓ x) EMIT
                                  (↓ "INCB" ↓X)
```

The general case might be:

```
Byte ↑ x → + Byte ↑ x Byte ↑ y EMIT (↓ "ADDB" ↓Y ↓X)
```

This method can use a single-pass bottom-up parser (for the IR) and attribute evaluation methods for the code generation.

10.7   Code Generator Generators

Code generator generators, also called automatic code generators, attempt to generate a code generator by abstracting the code generation process. This involves specification of machines, machine parts and operations. A number of such specifications have been studied.

Ideally, such specifications permit a complete and unambiguous description of the computer and its instruction set. To do so, they must make implicit assumptions about the structure of computers in general. A machine formalism is needed which is (1) sufficiently restrictive so code can be produced from an efficient algorithm but (2) permit specification of several typical computer architectures. Such descriptions have proved to be elusive, and compromises are usually made toward either (1) or (2).

We will discuss a few such models.

10.7.1   The ISP Model of Siewiorek, Bell and Newell (1982)

ISP stands for Instruction Set Processor Language and, as the name implies, describes computer instruction sets. An ISP specification describes data types, instructions, operations and processors. The data types define allowable data types such as integer or real data which can be stored.

Instructions are, themselves, data types. They describe the transformations, movement of data and transformations of data performed by instructions.

Operations also describe transformations on data.

Processors indicate the sequencing of instructions to be executed, memory definitions and address calculations.

10.7.2   The TDML Model of Glanville (1977)

The Target Machine Description Language, TDML, consists of four sections, the first of which is an optional listing for debugging. The remaining three sections list the registers, describe the IR nodes and describe the target machine's instruction set.

TDML allows the description of both registers and register classes. Two groups of registers may be specified: (1) *allocatable,* which are available for the register allocator to use, and (2) *dedicated*, which are reserved for specific functions such as instructions which require one of the operands to be in a particular register.

10.7.3   The PQCC Model (Wulf et al., 1980)

The model used in the Production Quality Compiler Compiler (PQCC) project is based on ISP.

In the PQCC model, machines are limited to a single processor which executes instructions stored in primary memory. The machine describes an instruction set processor which (repeatedly) fetches an instruction from primary memory, modifying the contents of the processor state.

The instruction set processor is defined by five components: (1) a storage base, (2) operand addressing, (3) machine operations, (4) data types and (5) construction fields and formats.

The storage base is an array of *length* words containing a (fixed) number of bits (the *width*). The *type* attribute indicates how the storage base is to be used. Typical values are *temporary* for storing values such as condition codes, *general purpose* for storing values, e.g., primary memory, and *reserved* to be used for registers such as the stack pointer or program counter.

Operand addressing specifies the *addressing mode* and any special purpose registers required. *Machine operations* represent the actual instructions and are associated with *assertions* which describe the changes made by an instruction.

10.8   Peephole Optimization

Peephole optimization is actually a family of optimizations that looks at a small number of lines of output code, looking for a pattern. It is so easy to do many of these that it is not unreasonable to put out poor code initially. It simplifies the code generation phase. Compiler designers look at the code produced when a compiler is up and running. This is called *profiling*. As they find new patterns actually produced, they keep adding optimization routines.

10.8.1   Unnecessary Loads

Consider the following code sequence:

```
STORE REG1,A
LOAD A,Reg2
```

Clearly, A is still in a register and there is no need to reload it into register 2.

10.8.2   Branch (to a) (around a) Branch

Many times compilers produce code that branches to another branch. Consider the following embedded CASE statements and the branches produced by a simple code generator:

Line Source	Output Code
50 WHILE a DO	50:
51 BEGIN	
...	
61 CASE i OF	
62 0: IF b THEN	
63 x := 1 ;	
64 ELSE	64: BRANCH 66
65 x := 2 ;	
66 {end case i = 0}	66: BRANCH 142
67 1:	
...	
81 4: CASE j OF	
...	
89 2: IF b THEN	
90 x := 0 ;	
91 ELSE	91: BRANCH 93
92 x := 1 ;	
93 {end case j =2 }	93: BRANCH 121
...	
120 end; {case j}	
121 {end case i = 4}	121: BRANCH 142
...	
141 end; {case i}	
142 end; {while a}	142: BRANCH 50

Just looking at the BRANCHes, we see:

```
50:
64: BRANCH 66
66: BRANCH 142
91: BRANCH 93
93: BRANCH 121
121: BRANCH 142
142: BRANCH 50
```

If we fully eliminated the indirect jumps, it would look like this:

```
50:
64: BRANCH 50
66: BRANCH 50
91: BRANCH 50
93: BRANCH 50
121: BRANCH 50
142: BRANCH 50
```

10.8.3   Cross-Jumping

IF-THEN-ELSE statements often produce almost duplicate code within the THEN and ELSE clauses. Consider the following:

```
IF Condition THEN
   A[I] := x + 1
ELSE
   A[I] := y + 1
```

The output code differs by only 1 load. We can perform that load and then execute the rest of the instructions: ADDing 1 and assigning to A[I]. This can be seen pictorially where Test is the code for the condition:

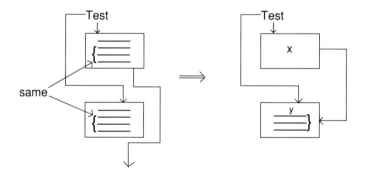

In the right-most picture the identical code is written only once.

10.8.4   Recognizing Special Instructions or Modes

Instructions that ADD one can often be replaced by an increment (for machines that have an increment instruction)

```
ADD #1,Reg2
```

may be substituted with

```
INCREMENT Reg2
```

Sometimes instructions can be combined by looking for the longest number of operators that can be turned into a single instruction. For example,

```
ADD Reg1,Reg2
MOVE Reg2,A
```

can be changed on some machines to

```
ADD Reg1,Reg2,A
```

Clearly, these cases are both source language dependent and machine dependent.

10.9 Summary

Code generation translates the intermediate representation of a program to executable code, while symbol table information is often translated to the storage allocation directives of a machine. The resulting instructions should be space and time efficient. Since resources such as registers are limited, choices are made when there is more than one way to perform the same computation.

A statement by statement code generator tends to produce poor code, where by "good" code we mean code that executes fast or takes up less space. To produce better code, code generation avoids extra computation, reusing computed values (common subexpressions) if reuse is less expensive than recomputing.

Further efficiency can be achieved by avoiding extra loads, unnecessary stores, avoidable register-to-register moves, and special instructions.

A good code generator *design*, like all software, is easier to implement, easier to test, and easier to maintain.

10.10 Related Reading

Aho, A. V., M. Ganapathi, and S. W. K. Tjiang. 1989. Code Generation Using Tree Matching and Dynamic Programming, *ACM TOPLAS*, 11(4):491–516.

Akin, T. A. and R. J. LeBlanc. 1982. The Design and Implementation of a Code Generation Tool, *Software-Practice and Experience*, 12:1027–1041.

Balachandran, A., D. M. Dhamdhere and S. Biswas. 1990. Efficient Retargetable Code Generation Using Bottom-Up Tree Pattern Matching, *Computer Languages*, 15(3).

Bernstein, D., M. Columbic, Y. Mansour, R. Pinter, D. Goldin, H. Krawczyk and I. Nahson. 1989. Spill Code Minimization Techniques for Optimizing Compilers, *SIGPLAN Notices*, 25(7).

Briggs., P. K. Cooper, K. Kennedy, and L. Torczon. 1989. Coloring Heuristics for Register Allocation, *SIGPLAN Notices*, 25(7).

Cattell, R. G. G. 1980. Automatic Derivation of Code Generators from Machine Descriptions, *ACM TOPLAS*, 2(2).

Chaitin, G. J., et al. 1981. Register Allocation via Coloring, *Computer Languages* 6:47–57.

Chow, F. C. 1988. Minimizing Register Usage Penalties at Procedure Calls, *SIGPLAN Notices*, 23(7).

Dhamdhere, D. M. 1990. A Usually Linear Algorithm for Register Assignment Using Edge Placement of Load and Store Instructions, *Computer Languages*, 15(2).

Ganapathi, M. J. and C. N. Fischer. 1983. Automatic Compiler Code Generation and Reusable Machine-Dependent Optimization—A Revised Bibliography, *ACM SIGPLAN Notices*, 18(4):27–34.

Ganapathi, M. J. and C. N. Fischer. 1984. Attributed Linear Intermediate Representations for Retargetable Code Generators, *Software-Practice and Experience*, 14(4):347–364.

Ganapathi, M. J. and C. N. Fischer. 1985. Affix Grammar Driven Code Generation, *ACM TOPLAS*, 7(4):560–599.

Ganapathi, M. J., J. L. Hennessy and C. N. Fischer. 1982. Retargetable Compiler Code Generation, *Computing Surveys*, 14(4):573–592.

Glanville, R. S. 1977. A Machine Independent Algorithm for Code Generation and Its Use in Retargetable Compilers, Ph.D. thesis, Dept. of EE and CS, Univ. of California, Berkeley.

Glanville, R. S. and S. L. Graham. 1978. *A New Method for Compiler Code Generation,* POPL Conference, 231–240.

Graham, S. L. 1980. Table-Driven Code Generation, *IEEE Computer*, August.

Graham, S. L. Code Generation and Optimization, in *Methods and Tools for Compiler Construction* (B. Lorho, ed.), Cambridge University Press.

Gupta, R., M. L. Soffa and G. Steele. 1989. Register Allocation via Clique Separators, *SIGPLAN Notices*, 24(7).

Horspool, R. N. and A. Scheunemann. 1985. Automating the Selection of Code Templates, *Software-Practice and Experience*, 15(5).

Keller, W. 1991. Automated Generation of Code Using Backtracking Parsers for Attribute Grammars, *SIGPLAN Notices*, 26(2):109–117.

Knuth, D. E. 1971. An Empirical Study of FORTRAN Programs, *Software Practice and Experience*, 1:105–133.

Lemone, K. A. 1985. *Assembly Language and System Programming for the IBM-PC and Compatibles*, Boston: Little, Brown.

Lemone, K. A. and M. E. Kaliski. 1987. *Assembly Language Programming for the VAX-11*, Boston: Little, Brown.

Siewiorek, D. P., G. C. Bell and A. Newell. 1982. *Computer Structures: Principles and Examples*, New York: McGraw-Hill, 1982.

Wulf et al. 1980. An Overview of the Production Quality Compiler-Compiler Project, *IEEE Computer* 13(8):38–49.

EXERCISES

1. (a) Using Belady's algorithm from Section 10.1.5 and the string

    uvwxuxvxw

show a register use sequence, assuming only two registers are available.

(b) Change the algorithm to the past tense and remove those variables which have not been used for the longest time.

2. (a) Create an abstract syntax tree for

$$(a + b) * (a - b) / ((c + d) * (c - d))$$

(b) Use the quick 'n dirty code generation algorithm from Example 3 to generate assembly language code.

(c) Label it using the labeling algorithm of Section 10.4 (assuming at least 1 of the 2 operands is to reside in a register) with the minimal number of registers needed to compute it.

(d) Using the code generation algorithm from Section 10.4, generate code for your tree

(i) Assuming there are 10 registers available

(ii) Assuming there are 2 registers available

3. Consider the following intermediate representation for code to multiply two matrices together:

```
        I := 1
        GOTO TestI
ILoop:  J := 1
        GOTO TestJ
JLoop:  C[I,J] := 0
        K := 1
        GOTO TestK
KLoop:  T1 := A[I,K] * B[K,J]
        T2 := C[I,J] + T1
        C[I,J] := T2
        K := K + 1
TestK:  IF K ≤ N GOTO KLoop
        J := J + 1
TestJ:  IF J ≤ N GOTO JLoop
        I := I + 1
TestI:  IF I ≤ N GOTO ILoop
```

Translate this into assembly language code:

(a) Using the templates from Section 10.3.1.

(b) By extending the algorithms in Section 10.4 (to handle IF's and loops)

4. Perform peephole optimization on the code produced in Example 1.

5. Perform peephole optimization on the code produced in Example 3.

6. Perform peephole optimization on the following, showing each step separately:

```
IF 5 > 0 THEN GOTO L1
    GOTO L2
L1: I := I + 1
L3: IF I > 5 GOTO L4
```

```
         GOTO L5
L4:  T1 := I * 1
     X := X + T1
     I := I + 1
     GOTO L3
L5:  GOTO L6
L2:  X := 0
L6:
```

7. Consider the following expression (Knuth, 1971):

```
C[I * N + J] := ((A + X) * y + 2 * 768 + ((L - M) * (-K)))/Z
```

(a) Show the AST representation of this and label each node with the minimal number of registers needed to compute it, assuming temporary results are kept in registers.

(b) Give the target code which uses the minimal number of registers, again assuming temporary results are kept in registers. Use the following instruction forms:

```
i.    R := M
ii.   M := R
iii.  Ri := Ri op Rj
iv.   Ri := Ri op M
```

plus the operator @ which means "address of" and indirection (Ri) which fetches the value whose address is stored in Ri.

8. Section 10.3.1 showed some code generation templates for symbol table entries, assignment statements, expressions, IF-THEN-ELSE's, WHILE loops, and arrays. Write code templates for

(a) FOR loops

(b) REPEAT loops

(c) CASE statements

9. Write a greedy algorithm to perform register allocation by coloring.

10. (a) Draw the interference graph for the program of Example 1.

(b) Find the minimal number of registers which allow variables X, Y, Z, and D to be assigned to registers.

11. Repeat Exercise 2 for a machine which performs multiplications and divisions by using (a) a register pair and (b) a register pair which must be consecutively even and odd, that is R2-R3, but not R3-R4.

Compiler Project Part 7

Code Generation

The goal here is to generate code which you then assemble, link and run (probably using a debugger to see—and show your instructor—results):

```
AST's + Symbol Table → Code
```

This means that you MUST NOT add semantic actions to the YACC, or other generator, BNF to put out code. To avoid rereading and restructuring the AST and the symbol table, you can add a post processor to your main program after the parser has parsed and created, via semantic actions, the AST and symbol table. For example, using C and YACC, this might look (something) like:

```
#include whatever
main ()
{
  yyparse() ;
  Other stuff
  GenCode() ;
  Maybe other stuff
}
```

Perform some minimal register allocation.

The following order is suggested for doing the assignment. Print out each one of these steps as you go along in case you never get the next step working.

A simple working code generator is worth more than a sophisticated nonworking one.

Step 1 Compile a sequence of assignment statements whose right-hand sides are expressions (start with just copy statements), and run the first program with just local names. Run other programs of your own making.

Step 2 Compile programs that include IF's and WHILE's using the first three programs of previous assignments and some of your own as input.

Step 3 Add some object-oriented features. For example, add class declarations to the first three programs. Send a meaningful message within the action part. Use imagination, but make the programs "useful".

Step 4 Run all previous test programs, changing them where necessary to get meaningful results.

Step 5 (*throwing down the gauntlet*) Write an object-oriented Quicksort program, declaring appropriate classes, instantiating (array?) objects and sending messages to get things done.

Hand in (at a minimum)

```
{Program-to-be-compiled
AST and Symbol Table
Assembly language code (commented if possible)
Debugger "Log" file}+
Plus your Code Generation program
```

Some of you may have already turned this project into a nice "package". If you want to include other outputs, say from LEX, that is okay. In fact, if you have time, it should be nicely packaged and documented, etc., but this is an extra.

This project is probably worth bringing to your next job interview, raise review, etc. Much of what we have done (in terms of an evolving language) is just what goes on in compiler projects.

11

Production-Quality Compilers

11.0 Introduction

Production-quality is a term used by compiler designers which has many definitions, depending on the environment for which a compiler is intended.

Many compiler designers would say that a compiler is production-quality if it implements all the features in the language, puts out good code and has good error diagnostics and recovery (Kukol, 1990). The cost here is in compiler performance, so this is not a good definition in terms of compiler performance. We will discuss features and techniques separately, pointing out their assets and liabilities. This will be especially important if "production-quality" means small and fast, and we will mention separately such features and techniques.

First, we list some techniques for the design process itself.

11.1 A Compiler as a Software Project

A compiler is a special type of large software project. Allen (1990) lists the following as phases of the compiler construction life cycle:

1. Specification Often, a compiler is designed from a language document. This document may change or may need to be changed as the project continues. Specifications of compile speed, produced code and space limitations must be considered.

2. Design Compilers may be bootstrapped from other compilers. They may use tools for many of their parts. Portability and retargetability need to be considered early in the design phase. Good interfaces are important. Key utilities such as node generators, tree-walk routines, printing utilities, etc. must be identified. These include the various tables to be used: symbol tables, type tables, label tables, most of which need to be accessed dynamically and read more than they are written to. Various intermediate representations may be designed.

3. Groundwork It is very important to build the right tools first, before building the compiler. Such tools may include a simulator if the hardware is new, since the compiler may need to be debugged before the hardware is ready. Other tools and utilities should identify and record clearly the various versions, centralize debugging and memory allocation, and identify the various compiler switches and listing utilities. Validation and testing programs should be assembled. A profiler should be created and used throughout the compiler creation life cycle. One should be prepared to measure everything.

4. Implementation   Steps 1 to 3 will lay out the compiler to be implemented. Coding standards will ease the assembling of the modules. Debugging must be built in. A centralized error processor saves work in the long run.

5. Maintenance   A large programming language compiler may be maintained for years and involve more person-hours than any of the other phases. Again, good tools, clear interfaces and good built-in debugger facilities, as well as coordinated bug reports, can aid this process.

6. Improvement   It is important to recognize early in the design process that improvements will be necessary. Techniques include a flexible framework that eases extensions.

11.2   Features, Techniques and Tradeoffs

In the remainder of this section, we discuss the standard phases. (We already know they may be merged.)

11.2.1   Scanning

For most languages—FORTRAN is a vivid exception—scanning is simple and requires little to no backtracking. Regular expressions can be designed and a tool used, or even better (say most compiler designers), a scanner itself can be written rather than generated. It has proved to be a better method than table-driven techniques. For FORTRAN, it may facilitate things to reuse a scanner from another system or even to buy one.

It is also best to keep the scanner simple, letting later phases do more work. This applies, in particular, to symbol table creation. A (hashed!) name table may be created during scanning, but the true symbol table is best created during semantic analysis, when names may be resolved. For example, Ada array references have the same syntax as function calls and can be distinguished only after declarations have been processed.

Lexical analysis is a good example of software that can be fine-tuned by writing some of the routines in assembler.

11.2.2   Parsing

The parsing method must be decided (see the summary to Chapter 5). If the parser is to be built from the BNF in a language design that is not LL(1), then LR(1) (LALR(1), more specifically) is the method of choice. Good error recovery is a difficult part of this phase, no matter what parsing method is chosen. Again, simple is better and parsing should consist of syntax analysis; static checking and other semantic analyses can be pushed off to the semantic analysis phase.

Again, for a small, fast compiler, the advice may be just the opposite: syntax analysis should be tightly coupled with semantic analysis.

11.2.3   Semantic Analysis

Semantic analysis is the bridge between parsing and code generation. The levels and number of intermediate representations depend upon the goals of the compiler. Trees are simplest; graphs may be required for serious optimizations.

For small and fast, it is desirable to minimize the number of visits to each node; for example Sethi-Ullman numbering may be done as the abstract syntax tree is generated. Perhaps the object code may be emitted directly, although this will result in poorer quality code.

11.2.4   Optimization

Some languages, such as FORTRAN, really require optimization to produce even moderately efficient code. For other languages, it may be a toss-up, and something to be added during the improvements phase of the compiler life cycle. The other factor which promotes the need for, and newer techniques for, optimization is the newer machine architectures (e.g., RISC machines). Techniques for optimizing for such machines will be discussed in Chapter 12.

Aggressive optimizations are also a major source of bugs in a compiler.

11.2.5   Code Generation

Table-driven techniques increase the portability of the compiler, but often a few machine-dependent features can make the code generator more efficient. Code generation requires a balance between flexibility and the use of known machine details.

Although most of this book has presumed generation of assembly language, most compiler people would maintain that generating assembler code is not a production-quality technique.

Debugger interaction with highly optimized code is difficult unless the compiler leaves a clear trail of the changes made. Standardization of object file formats has been proposed, but not accepted yet.

11.2.6   Tradeoffs

Portability, including retargetability and rehostability, may be traded off for simplicity and efficiency. Aggressive optimization may be traded off for compiler stability and performance of the compiler itself.

Small and fast compilers are required for microcomputers. They require fewer functional interfaces, fewer passes and much mixing of phases, and an avoidance of data transformations, that is, a tighter coupling. The tradeoff is a software package that is more difficult to maintain.

11.2.7   Other System Software

The compiler does not execute in isolation. As well as the operating system, the compiler needs to be aware of the assembler, linker, debugger, runtime systems and libraries, and perhaps also a profiler, a graphical tool and a simulator.

11.2.8   Portability

Compilers are such large programs that the ability to move a compiler from one machine to another is a definite asset. Some software companies build compilers for one or two languages and then stay in business by "porting" them to and marketing them for other machines.

In addition to other machines, sometimes a compiler is to be ported from one environment or operating system to another. As UNIX became more widely used, much software was "retargeted" for this environment.

The issues in retargeting are often code generation issues: different addressing modes, different operations, a different number of registers and run-time library all need to be addressed. Memory layout may be quite different. Object code formats are different for different machines.

11.2.9 Benchmarks

Benchmark programs measure the efficiency of compilers (and machines). Some well-known benchmark programs are Whetstone (Curnow and Wichmann, 1976; Weicker, 1990) and Dhrystone (Weicker, 1984, 1990). Whetstone was developed for scientific computing applications and is heavy in floating-point operations. Dhrystone was developed for non-numerical applications and is heavy in string operations.

Another frequently used measurement is MIPS (Millions of Instructions Per Second). Without a base value to compare to, however, this becomes "Meaningless Indication of Processor Speed". For example, a one statement instruction on a non-RISC processor might require four statements on a RISC machine; it would be incorrect, if the execution speed were the same, to say that the RISC machine is four times as fast.

In addition, language-specific benchmarks are common. This is especially true of languages like Ada (Clapp et al., 1988). Measurement of the performance of specific language features is useful in specific applications.

More useful benchmark programs are those which are actually used, especially if the environment in which the compiler is to be run is known. For example, YACC is a compute-intensive program and is often run as a benchmark program. Other familiar software such as $L_A T_E X$, troff, awk and various compilers are often used. Special programs such as the Sieve of Eratosthenes and Quicksort are sometimes used since they can be recoded into whatever language is being compiled.

11.2.10 Validations

Asserting that a compiler is correct is becoming more formal. Validation programs for older languages such as FORTRAN and Cobol evolved after the languages were implemented. Ada was one of the first languages to be designed with the provision that compilers for it must be able to run specifically designed validation programs.

11.3   Run-Time Storage Management

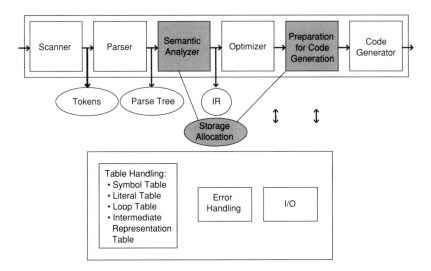

The previous sections of this book presume that assembly language code is to be generated by our compiler. When this is done, we need not worry about allocating space for program quantities. The assembler and other system software take care of this. Production-quality compilers (usually) do not put out assembly language code. Instead, they emit object code directly. This text does not discuss object code formats for particular machines. Instead, we discuss how the compiler facilitates the storage of information that is to take place at run-time. All of these actions could be considered as part of either the semantic analysis phase or as preparation for code generation.

Values are assigned to variables at execution time, but it is the compiler, at compile time, which performs the necessary bookkeeping so that this happens smoothly.

If we consider a program as a sequence of "unit" calls (with the main program being the first unit), then we can see immediately some of the issues. Suppose a variable, declared to be of type integer, is assigned an integer-sized space in the machine. What happens if this unit is a procedure called recursively? Clearly, there must be more than one such space allocated for such a variable.

In this chapter, we will proceed from simple languages (simple storage-wise!) like FORTRAN, which do not allow recursion to languages that allow recursion, and data structures like pointers whose storage requirements change during execution.

11.3.1   Compile-Time Decisions

Decisions made at compile time include where to put information and how to get it. These are the same decisions made about symbol tables (see Exercise 5), but here the information is different. For symbol tables, we are concerned about information that is known at compile time, in particular the symbol's class. Here, we are concerned about information *not* entirely known at compile time, such as a particular symbol's value or how many instances there will be of a variable due to recursive calls.

11.3.2   Run-Time Information

Storage must be allocated for user-defined data structures, variables, and constants. The compiler also facilitates procedure linkage; that is, the return address for a procedure call must be stored somewhere.

This can be thought of as *binding* a value to a storage location and the binding can be thought of as a mapping:

> Source Language $\rightarrow$ Target Machine

Thus, although some of the later optimization phase is independent of the machine, the run-time storage algorithms are somewhat machine dependent.

11.3.3   Unit Activation

Many of the compile-time decisions for run-time storage involve procedure calls. For each procedure or function, including the main program, the compiler constructs a *program unit* to be used at execution time. A program unit is composed of a *code segment,* which is the code to be executed, and an *activation record,* which is the information necessary to execute the code segment.

A code segment is fixed since it consists of (machine code) instructions, while the activation record information is changeable since it references the variables which are to receive values.

11.3.4   Activation Records

The information in an activation record varies according to the language being compiled. An activation record can be of a fixed or variable size.

A typical activation record contains space to record values for local data and parameters or references to such space. It also contains the return location in the code so that execution can resume correctly when the procedure finishes.

The term *offset* is used to describe the relative position of information in an activation record, that is, its position relative to the beginning of the activation record.

11.3.5   Language Issues

Different languages have different needs at run-time. For example, the standard version of FORTRAN *permits* all decisions to be made at compile-time. (It doesn't *require* this to be done.)

We say that FORTRAN-like languages have *static* storage allocation. This means that at compile-time *all* decisions are made about where information will reside at run-time:

11.3.6   Static Storage Allocation

Because FORTRAN typifies the issues for static storage allocation, it will be used as the example here. For FORTRAN and other languages which allow static storage allocation, the amount of storage required to hold each variable is fixed at translation time.

Such languages have no nested procedures or recursion and thus only one instance of each *name* (the same identifier may be used in different contexts, however).

In FORTRAN each procedure or function, as well as the main program and a few other program structures not discussed here, may be compiled separately and associated with an activation record that can be entirely allocated by the compiler.

Example 1 shows the skeleton of a FORTRAN program and its storage allocation.

EXAMPLE 1   Static storage example

Consider the following outline of a FORTRAN program, where statements beginning with *C* represent comments.

```
C Main Program
  ...
  Read (*,X)
  ...
C Function ...
  FUNCTION ...
  ...
C Subroutine ...
  SUBROUTINE ...
  ...
```

For each program unit such as the main program, a function or a subroutine (procedure), there is a code segment and an activation record. Figure 1 is a picture of what the run-time system might look like for the program skeleton of Example 1:

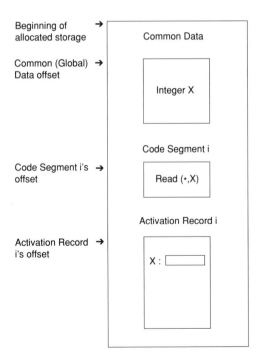

Figure 1

Figure 2 shows *X*'s offset within the activation record:

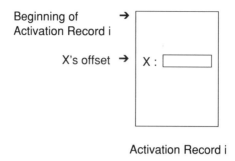

Activation Record i

Figure 2

Notice that everything except the beginning of the allocated storage is known at compile-time: the position (offset) of the activation record within the data area and even *X* 's position (offset) within the activation record for its unit. The only decision to be made at run-time (and often made by the system linker) is where to put the entire data structure.

In static storage allocation, variables are also said to be *static* because their offset in the run-time system structure can be completely determined at compile time.

11.3.7   Activation Records for Languages that Support Recursion

For languages that support recursion, it is necessary to be able to generate different data spaces since the data for each recursive call are kept in the activation record.

Such activation records are typically kept on a *stack*.

When there is more than one recursive call which has not yet terminated, there will be more than one activation record, perhaps for the same code segment.

An extra piece of information must thus be stored in the activation record—the address of the previous activation record. This pointer is called a *dynamic link* and points to the activation record of the calling procedure.

Languages such as Algol, Pascal, Modula, C and Ada all allow recursion and require at least the flexibility of a stack-based discipline for storage.

Example 2 shows a program and its stack of activation records when the program is executing at the point marked by the asterisks. The program is not in any particular language, but is pseudocode.

EXAMPLE 2   Activation record structure for a recursive call

```
PROGRAM Main
  LOCAL a,b
  PROCEDURE P(PARAMETER x)
    LOCAL p1,p2
  BEGIN {P}
    Call P(p2) ***
  END {P}
```

```
BEGIN {Main}
  Call P(a)
END {Main}
```

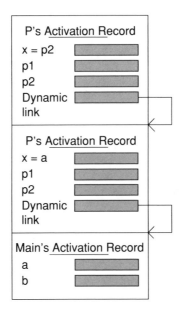

In Example 2, *main*'s activation record contains space to store the values for the variables *a* and *b*. The activation record stacked on top of the activation record for main represents the activation record for the (first) call to *P*. *P*'s parameter *x* has actual value *a*, and there is space for its value, as well as space for the local variables *p1* and *p2*. The address of the previous activation record is stored in *dynamic link*.

On the other hand, the *amount* of storage required for each variable *is* known at translation time, so, like FORTRAN, the *size* of the activation record and a variable's offset is known at translation (compile) time. Since recursive calls require that more than one activation record for the same code segment be kept, it is not possible, as in FORTRAN, to know the offset of the activation record itself at compile-time. Variables in these languages are termed *semistatic*.

11.3.8 Activation Records for Languages that Support Block Structure

Block-structured languages allow units to be nested. Most commonly, it is subprograms (procedures) that are nested, but languages such as Algol and C allow a new unit to be created, and nested, merely by enclosing it with BEGIN-END or similar constructs.

The unit within which a variable is "known" and has a value is called its *scope*. For many languages a variable's scope includes the unit where it is defined and any contained units, but not units that contain the unit where the variable is defined.

During execution, block-structured languages cause a new complication since a value may be assigned or accessed for a variable declared in an "outer" unit. This is a problem because the activation record for the unit currently executing is not necessarily the activation record where the value is to be stored or found.

A new piece of information must be added to the activation record to facilitate this access. Pointers called *static links* point to the activation records of units where variables, *used* in the current procedure, are *defined*. *Uplevel addressing* refers to the reference in one unit of a variable defined in an outer unit. A sequence of static links is called a *static chain*.

Example 3 makes two changes to the program of Example 2. The variables *a* and *b* are now global to the program, and procedure *P* references variable *a*. An additional field, the static link, is shown in *P*'s activation record.

EXAMPLE 3   Block structure

```
PROGRAM Main
  GLOBAL a,b
  PROCEDURE P(PARAMETER x)
    LOCAL p1,p2
  BEGIN {P}
    ...a...
    Call P(p2) ***
  END {P}
BEGIN {Main}
  Call P(a)
END {Main}
```

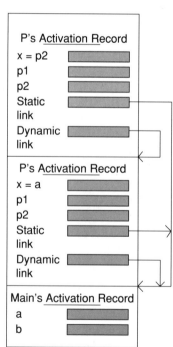

In Example 3, the static link points from the activation records for *P* to that for *Main* since *P* is nested within *Main*.

Once again though, the actual size of the activation record is known at compile-time.

11.3.9   Activation Records Whose Size Is Known at Unit Activation

There are language constructs where neither the size of the activation record nor the position of the information within the activation record is known until the unit begins execution.

One such construct is the *dynamic array* construct. Here, a unit can declare an array to have dimensions that are not fixed until run-time. Example 4 shows the program from Examples 2 and 3, with such a dynamic array declaration and its activation record structure

EXAMPLE 4   Dynamic arrays

```
PROGRAM Main
  GLOBAL a,b
  PROCEDURE P(PARAMETER x)
    LOCAL p1,p2
    ARRAY P3:[1:a]
  BEGIN {P}
    ...a...
    Call P(p2)
  END {P}
BEGIN {Main}
  ...
  Call P(a)
END {Main}
```

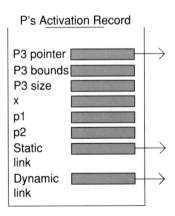

P's Activation Record

In Example 4, the dimensions for *P3* are known when procedure *P* is activated (called).

Clearly, if the values for array *P3* are to be kept in an activation record for *P3*, the size of the record cannot be fixed at translation time. If *a* is given a value within *P*, as well as within *Main*, it is possible that the activation record for *P* will be a different size for each invocation.

What can be created at compile-time is space in the activation record to store the size and bounds of the array. A place containing a pointer to the beginning of the array can also be created (this is necessary if there is more than one such dynamic structure). At execution time, the record can be fully expanded to the appropriate size to contain all the values or the values can be kept somewhere else, say on a heap (described below).

Variables, like the dynamic arrays just described, are called *semidynamic variables*. Space for them is allocated by reserving storage in the activation record for a *descriptor* of the semidynamic variable. This descriptor might be a pointer to the storage area as well as the upper and lower bounds of each dimension.

At run-time the storage required for semidynamic variables is allocated. The dimension entries are entered in the descriptor, the actual size of semidynamic variable is evaluated and the activation record is expanded to include space for the variable or a call is made to the operating system for space and the descriptor pointer is set to point to the area just allocated.

11.3.10 Activation Records with Dynamically Varying Size

There are languages that contain constructs whose values vary in size, not just as a unit is invoked, as in the previous section, but during the unit's execution. Pascal (and other language) pointers, flexible arrays (whose bounds change during execution), strings in languages such as Snobol, and lists in Lisp are a few examples. These all require *on demand* storage allocation, and such variables are called *dynamic variables*.

Example 5 shows the problems encountered with such constructs.

EXAMPLE 5   Dynamic variables

```
PROGRAM Main
  GLOBAL a,b
  DYNAMIC p4
  PROCEDURE P(PARAMETER x)
    LOCAL p1,p2
  BEGIN {P}
    NEW(p4)
    Call P(p2)  ***
  END {P}
BEGIN {Main}
  Call P(a)
END {Main}
```

In Example 5, notice that *p4* is declared in *Main*, but not used until procedure *P*. Suppose that the program is executing at the point where the asterisks are shown, using the stack of activation record structure as in the previous examples. Where should space for $p4$'s value be allocated?

P's activation record is on top of the stack. If space for $p4$ is allocated in P, then when P finishes, this value will go away (incorrectly). Allocating space for $p4$ in *main* is possible since the static link points to it, but it would require reshaping P's activation record, a messy solution since lots of other values (e.g., the dynamic links) would need to be adjusted.

The solution here is not to use a stack, but rather a data structure called a *heap*.

Heap

A heap is a block of storage within which pieces are allocated and freed in some relatively unstructured way.

Heap storage management is needed when a language allows the creation, destruction or extension of a data structure at arbitrary program points. It is implemented by calls to the operating system to create or destroy a certain amount of storage.

We will discuss more about heaps for Lisp-like programming languages.

11.3.11 Activation Records for Concurrent Units

Languages such as Ada, which allow concurrent execution of program units, pose additional storage allocation problems in that *each* concurrently executing unit (*tasks* in Ada) requires a stack-like storage.

One approach is to use a heap. Still another solution is to use a data structure called a *cactus stack*.

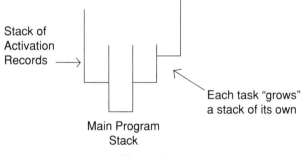

Stack of
Activation
Records ⟶

Each task "grows"
a stack of its own

Main Program
Stack

Figure 3

11.3.12 Storage Allocation for Lisp-like Languages

Lisp is a programming language whose primary data structure is a list. During execution, lists can grow and shrink in size and thus are implemented using a heap data structure.

Although we refer explicitly to Lisp here, we could equally well be discussing Snobol, a string-oriented language, or any other language that requires data to be created and destroyed during program execution.

In Lisp-like languages, a new element may be added to an existing list structure at any point, requiring storage to be allocated. A heap pointer, say, *Hp,* is set to point to the next free element on the heap. As storage is allocated, this pointer is continually updated. Calls to operating system routines manage this allotment.

Certainly, if storage is continually allocated and not recovered, the system may soon find itself out of space. There are two ways of recovering space: *explicitly* and *garbage collection,* a general technique used in operating systems. We will discuss these two as they relate to Lisp.

Explicit Return of Storage

Consider the list α in Figure 4, where each element contains two fields: the information field and a field containing a pointer to the next element of the list. The element α, itself, points to (contains the address of) the first element in the list.

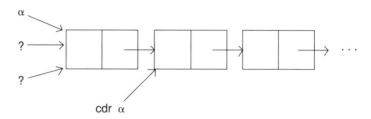

Figure 4

In LISP, an operator called (for historical reasons) *cdr,* given a pointer to one element in a list, returns a pointer to the next element on the list.

The question is whether or not *cdr* should cause the pointer α to be returned to the heap.

If α is the only pointer and *cdr doesn't* return it to the heap, then it becomes "garbage" (a technical term whose meaning should be clear!).

However, if *cdr* does return it and other pointers (shown as "?" in the picture above) do exist, then they become *dangling references*; they no longer point to α because it no longer exists.

Unfortunately, it is difficult to know, although some creative (and time consuming!) bookkeeping could keep track. The alternative is to allow garbage to be created and periodically to "clean up", a method called *garbage collection.*

Garbage Collection

When the garbage collection method is used, garbage is allowed to be created. Thus there is no dangling reference problem.

When the heap becomes exhausted (empty), a garbage collection mechanism is invoked to identify and recover the garbage. The following describes a garbage collection algorithm. It presumes that each element in the system has an extra bit called a "garbage collection bit" initially set to "on" for all elements.

Algorithm

Garbage Collection

Step 1. Mark "active" elements, that is, follow all active pointers, turning "off" the garbage collection bits for these active elements.

Step 2. Collect garbage elements, that is, perform a simple sequential scan to find elements with garbage bit on and return them to the heap.

11.3.13 Storage Allocation for Arrays

The previous sections have discussed storage allocation "in the large", that is, the general activation record mechanisms necessary to facilitate assignment of data to variables.

Here, we discuss one issue "in the small", that of computing the offset for an element in an array. Other data structures such as records can be dealt with similarly (see Exercise 1).

Computation of Array Offsets

Array references can be simple, such as

```
A[I]
```

or complex, such as

```
A[I - 2,C[U]]
```

In either case the variables can be used in an equation that can be set up (but not evaluated) at compile-time.

We will do this first for an array whose first element is assumed to be at $A[1,1,1, \ldots ,1]$.

That is, given an array declaration

```
A: ARRAY[d₁, d₂, ... dₖ] OF some type
```

what is the address of

```
A[i₁,i₂, ... iₖ]
```

It is easiest to think of this for the one- or two-dimensional case. For two dimensions, what is the offset for

```
A[i₁,i₂], given a declaration
A: ARRAY[d₁,d₂] OF some type
```

By offset, we mean the distance from the base (beginning) of the array which we will call base(A).

To reach $A[i_1,i_2]$ from base(A), one must traverse all the elements in rows 1 through $i_1 - 1$ plus all the columns up to i_2 in row i_1. There are d_2 elements in each of the i_1 rows; thus, $A[i_1,i_2]$'s offset is:

```
(i₁ - 1) * d₂ + i₂
```

The absolute address is

```
base(A) + (i₁ - 1) * d₂ + i₂
```

For k-dimensions the address is:

$$\text{base(A)} + (((((i_1 - 1)\ d_2 + (i_2 - 1)) \star d_3 + (i_3 - 1))$$
$$\star\ d_4 + \ldots) \star d_k + i_k$$

or

$$\text{base(A)} + (i_1 - 1) \star d_2 d_3 . d_k + (i_2 - 1) \star d_3 \ldots d_k + \ldots$$
$$+ (i_{k-1} - 1) \star d_k + i_k$$

The second way is better for the optimization phase because the sum of indices is multiplied by constants, and these constants can be computed at compile time via constant computation and constant propagation.

In the next section, we discuss an implementation method using attribute grammars. This was touched upon in Chapter 6.

Computation of Array Offsets Using Attribute Grammars

Consider the following grammar for array references:

```
Name          → Id
Name          → Id[Subscripts]
Subscripts    → Id
Subscripts    → Subscripts , Id
```

We want to be able to attach attributes and semantic functions to these.

Example 6 shows a three-dimensional example and attributes *Dims*, *NDim* and *Offset*. *Dims* is an inherited attribute. It consults the symbol table at the node for the array name (*A* here) and fetches the values d_1, d_2, and d_3 which are stored there. These are handed down the tree and used in the computation of *Offset*, which is a synthesized attribute. Attribute *NDim* is a counter that counts the number of dimensions, presumably for error checking.

EXAMPLE 6   Calculation of $(I - 1) * d_2 * d_3 + (J - 1) * d_3 + K$

Consider the declaration:

```
A : ARRAY [d₁,d₂,d₃] OF some type
```

and the parse tree for the reference:

```
A[I,J,K]
```

with inherited attribute *Dims* shown descending the tree

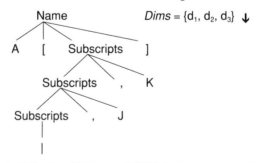

and synthesized attributes *NDim* and *OffSet* shown ascending the tree:

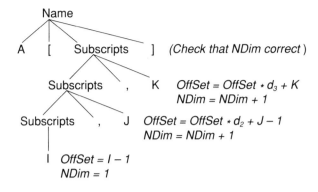

Exercise 3 asks the reader to write the semantic functions to compute the values for these attributes, while Exercise 4 suggests another way to write the grammar that will allow the attributes to be evaluated in one pass up the tree. This is material repeated from Chapter 6, so the reader may wish to refer back to that chapter.

The exercises ask the reader to consider other compile-time structures which have storage needs such as record.

In Sections 11.5 and 11.6, we describe a few compilers to see how a compiler in the real world has made the compromises described in this chapter (as well as other compromises).

11.4   Incremental Compiling

Many of the first language processors operated incrementally. A programmer typed a line and it was processed right through to execution. BASIC interpreters were (and are) designed for this model. More complex language constructs and needs for efficient translation lead to compilers and the decrease of these early incremental techniques.

Modern programming language environments, with syntax-directed editors and complex optimizations, have discovered a new need for incremental translation techniques. In general, it is wasteful to recompile an entire program when a small change has been made.

The high-level techniques described in Sections 8.7 and 9.5 are amenable to incremental processing. Many Ada compilers (see Section 11.6) also take advantage of recently developed techniques for incremental compilation. We will divide the incremental discussion here into front-end and back-end issues.

When programs consist of a number of separately compiled units, a unit may need to be recompiled, or partially recompiled, when a change is made to that unit or a change is made to to any unit in which the unit's identifiers are declared. A clever compiler [Tichy, 1986] can discover when a compilation is redundant.

11.4.1   Incremental Parsing

Ideally, incremental parsing would allow reparsing only the part of a program which has been changed in the course of editing or the parts of the program affected by the editing. Many syntax-directed editors parse and enforce syntax correctness by restricting changes to those which result in a syntactically correct parse tree.

Unfortunately, as we know from previous chapters, not all syntax issues can be incorporated into the context-free grammar (BNF). For example, enforcement of consistency between data declarations and uses is not expressible using BNF alone.

Attribute grammars, which allow a fuller range of expression, have proven useful for incremental parsing.

11.4.2   Incremental Semantic Analysis

Incremental semantic analysis, in particular incremental attribute evaluation, can aid in incremental parsing by propagating changes to attributes around the tree in just the affected area. The method is to make a change to an attribute and then use the semantic functions to update changes upward (for synthesized attributes) or downward (for inherited attributes) *just* until nodes are encountered where the values do not change.

The attributes which apply to use and definition of variables (see Chapter 6, Exercise 9 and Chapter 8, Section 7) are particularly amenable to this efficient recalculation.

11.4.3   Incremental Data Flow Analysis

Data flow solutions involve propagation of values until changes cease. Once a data flow analysis has been done, a change can be propagated around the control flow graph [Ryder and Paull, 1988] or parse tree [Rosen, 1977; Babich and Jazayeri, 1978] just until changes once again cease.

11.4.4   Incremental Optimization

Since optimization algorithms tend to act in passes, looking for templates to optimize, incremental updating of the data flow information tends to aid in incremental optimization. Alternatively, optimization algorithms may "call" the data flow calculation procedures and request that a data flow value be calculated (see Babich and Jazayeri, 1978) much as a parser calls the scanner, requesting that a new token be produced.

11.5   Compiler Example: Borland International's Turbo Pascal

Turbo Pascal is one of the compilers whose needs are described by the small but fast compiler techniques of Section 11.2.6.

Turbo Pascal supports the full range of standard Pascal as well as a few features of its own such as a byte data type, special array types, additional arithmetic operators, built-in strings and much more.

It is small because it was originally designed for the 86-family of computers with limited physical memory. In fact, it is designed to run in the absence of a hard disk if necessary.

Turbo Pascal is fast, processing more than 30,000 lines/minute on a two MIP (millions of hardware instructions per minute) machine. This translates to 15,000 lines/minute/MIP.

Memory management must deal with the 86-family's segmented architecture (see Lemone, 1986) and with limited operating services.

Turbo Pascal emphasizes environments and comes with its own editor and debugger.

Turbo Pascal does not follow the textbook structure of separate phases and modular design which would enhance portability, reliability and maintainability, although Turbo Pascal is quite reliable and has been ported to other machines. Such designs would be too large and too slow.

The scanner consumes about 25% of the compiler while the parser takes 30–40% and 30–40% is for code generation. The parser is recursive descent (thus contradicting the belief that recursive descent is not the method of choice for "serious" compilers). The semantic analysis phase is mixed with parsing and does not change to an intermediate representation.

Turbo Pascal has fewer functional interfaces, eliminates many passes and mixes phases.

Earlier versions of Turbo Pascal used a linear symbol table structure. Later versions use a more efficient structure.

Live variable analysis is limited to fewer than 16 variables on 16-bit versions of the 86-family and to 32 bits on the 32-bit versions, so that bit vectors may be used (see Chapter 8). Other optimizations include constant propagation, which is performed "on the fly" as the tree is built.

Turbo Pascal does not do error recovery. Because the environment is integrated, the user is put back into the editor when an error is encountered.

Because the original Turbo Pascal is written for the 86-family, whose architecture presents "unique problems", code generation must be aware of special purpose registers. When Turbo Pascal was ported to the 68000, the code generator was reduced by half.

To complete the non-textbook approach: the original Turbo Pascal was written entirely in assembler!

11.6   Compiler Example: Ada Compilers

There are many Ada compilers. Rather than describing one, some problems and features, in general, will be mentioned. Many Ada compilers are designed for special architectures, so much of the material in Chapter 12 applies to Ada compilers. The reference at the end of the chapter include more detailed reports on Ada compiler technology (see, in particular, Ganapathi and Mendal, 1989).

Ada is a complex language with difficult to implement constructs. It was designed by a committee over a period of years. An Ada compiler is not deemed official unless it passes a validation suite which was designed at the same time as the language was designed.

Ada is designed for separate compilation, that is, it is designed so that modules, called *packages,* may be compiled separately and then linked. Incremental compilation is supported by most Ada compilers in the recompilation of packages. Many compilers support incremental recompilation at the semantic analysis phase when a change is "local".

On multiprocessor systems, compiler phases, which are not dependent upon one another, may be compiled in parallel.

Most Ada systems consist of an environment of a syntax-directed and semantics-directed editors, a debugger, and other tools. The compiler is but one of the tools.

Ada is designed with its own high-level intermediate representation, Diana (Descriptive Intermediate Attributed Notation for Ada), and a lower level IR, called CGIR.

Type checking in Ada is an important part of the semantic analysis phase. Ada allows overloading of many constructs including functions and procedures (see Chapter 2). Ada also requires *strong typing*, that is, the type of a name must be resolved at compile time.

Optimization is especially important in Ada compilers since one of Ada's stated applications is in embedded systems, systems which often must run in real-time. Many optimizations are machine dependent; RISC machines in particular (see Chapter 12) present opportunities for optimizations.

11.7   Summary

A compiler is a large programming project, but a highly visible one, within a computer system. Like many large pieces of software, good tools and good design facilitate the entire process.

This chapter has also discussed data structures and techniques used by compilers to facilitate decisions to be made at run-time. Many of the data structures for run-time structures are the same as those for symbol tables; we could easily use a stack symbol table structure for block-structured languages. Language features such as recursion, block structure and dynamic variables influence the type of run-time system required.

If a program is to be translated to assembly language, the assembler's run-time system takes care of many of the issues discussed here (see Project Part 8, Option 1).

A translated program requires space for the code as well as for the static data, and any space needed for the stack or heap data.

Real-life compilers often make compromises with the textbook descriptions as illustrated by Turbo Pascal.

In Chapter 12, we will discuss specific compiler details for compilers for special architectures such as RISC machines.

11.8   Related Reading

Allen, R. 1990. *Putting It All Together*, SIGPLAN'90 Advanced Topics Tutorial, White Plains, New York.

Babich, W. A. and M. Jazayeri. 1978. The Method of Attributes for Data Flow Analysis, Part I: Exhaustive Analysis, and Part II: Demand Analysis, *Acta Informatica*, 10(3):245–272.

Ballance, R. A., J. Butcher, and S. L. Graham. 1988. *Grammatical Abstraction and Incremental Syntax Analysis in a Language-Based Editor*, Proceedings of the SIGPLAN 88 Conference on Programming Language Design and Implementation, Atlanta, 185–198.
    Recommends use of an abstract syntax for incremental parsing.

Birens, M. P. and M. L. Soffa. 1990. Incremental Register Allocation, *Software Practice and Experience*, 20(10).

Burke, M. 1990. *An Interval-Based Approach to Exhaustive and Incremental Interprocedural Data Flow Analysis*, 12(3).

Clapp, R. M., L. Duchesneau, R. A. Volz, T. N. Mudge and T. Schultze. 1988. Toward Real-Time Performance Benchmarks for Ada, *CACM*, 29(8):760–778.
  Recommends measuring performance of language features.

Conte, T. and W. Hwe. 1991. Benchmark Characterization, *Computer*, 24(1):48–56.

Curnow, H. J. and B. A. Wichmann. 1976. A Synthetic Benchmark, *Computer Journal*, 19:43–49.
  Describes the classic Whetstone benchmark. Measures computers and compilers efficiency with a number of scientific programs.

Demers, A., T. Reps, and T. Teitelbaum. 1981. *Incremental Evaluation for Attribute Grammars with Application to Syntax-Directed Editors*, Proceedings of the eighth annual Symposium on Principles of Programming Languages, Williamsburg, VA, Jan. 26–28, 105–116.
  Discusses the advantages of using attribute grammars to build syntax-directed editors to enforce syntax correctness incrementally.

Fleming, P. J. and J. J. Wallace. 1986. How Not to Lie with Statistics: the Correct Way to Summarize Benchmark Results, *CACM*, 29(30):218–221.
  Provides guidelines on using maximum, minimum, and deviations when reporting mean benchmark values.

Ganapathi, M. and G. O. Mendal. 1989. Issues in Ada Compiler Technology, *IEEE Computer*, 22(2):52–60.

Goodenough, J. B. 1986. *The Ada Compiler Validation Capability Implementors' Guide*, SofTech Inc., Waltham, MA.

Heymann, J. 1991. A Comprehensive Analytical Model for Garabage Collection Algorithms, *SIGPLAN Notices*, 26(8):50–59.

Holub, A. 1990. *Compiler Design in C*, Englewood Cliffs, NJ: Prentice-Hall, 1990.

Horowitz, S., T. Reps and D. Binkley. 1990. *Interprocedural Slicing Using Dependence Graphs*, 12(1):26–60.

Hudson, S. 1991. Incremental Attribute Evaluation: A Flexible Algroithm for Lazy Update, *ACM Transactions on Programming Languages and Systems*, 13(3):315–341.

Iturbide, J. and A. Valazquez. 1989 Formalization of the Control Stack, *SIGPLAN Notices*, 24(3):46–54.

Kukol, P. 1990. *Developing Small and Fast Production-Quality Compilers*, SIGPLAN'90 Advanced Topics Tutorial, White Plains New York.

Lemone, K. 1986. *Assembly Language and System Programming for the IBM-PC and Compatibles*, Boston: Little, Brown.

Morisson, R., M. P. Atkinson, A.L. Brown, and A. Dearle. 1988. Bindings in Persistent Programming Languages, *SIGPLAN Notices*, 23(4):27–34.

Murching, A. M. and Y. N. Srikant, Inc. 1989. *Attribute Evaluation Through Recursive Procedures*, 14(4).
  Presents an incremental evaluation technique similar to the (non-incremental) evaluation technique of Katayama described in Chapter 6.

Murtagh, T. 1991. An Improved Storage Management Scheme for Block Structured Languages, *ACM Transactions on Programming Languages and Systems,* 13(3):372–398.

Pollack, L. L. and M. L. Soffa. 1990. Incremental Global Optimizations for Faster Recompilation, *Proceedings of the 1990 IEEE International Conference on Computer Languages.*

Pollack, L. L. and M. L. Soffa. 1989. An Incremental Version of Iterative Data Flow Analysis, *IEEE Transactions on Software Engineering,* 15(12):1537–1549.

Reps, T., T. Teitelbaum. and A. Demers. 1983. Incremental Context-Dependent Analysis for Language-Based Editors, *ACM Transactions on Programming Languages and Systems,* 5(3):449–477.
Describes efficient techniques for modification of attribute values after program changes.

Rosen, B. 1977. High-Level Data Flow Analysis, *CACM,* 20(10):712–724.

Ryder, B. G. and M. C. Paull. 1988. Incremental Data-Flow Analysis Algorithms, *ACM Transactions on Programming Languages and Systems,* 10(1):1–50.
Presents algorithms which recalculate data flow solutions on only the part of the program affected.

Szafron, P. and R. Ng. 1990. *LexAGen: An Interactive Incremental Scanner Generator,* 20(5).

Tichy, W. F. 1986. Smart Recompilation, *ACM Transactions on Programming Languages and Systems,* 8(6):273-291.
Describes a method for reducing the set of modules that must be recompiled after a change.

Treadway, P. L. 1990. The Use of Sets as an Application Programming Technique, *SIGPLAN Notices,* 25(5):103-116.

Weicker, R. P. 1990. An Overview of Common Benchmarks, *IEEE Computer,* Dec:65–75.

Weicker, R. P. 1984. Dhrystone: A Synthetic Systems Programming Benchmark, *Communications of the ACM,* 27(10):1013–1030.

Wilson, P. 1991. Some Issues and Strategies in Heap Management and Memory Hierarchies, *SIGPLAN Notices,* 26(3).

Yellin, D. and R. Strom. 1991. INC: A Language for Incremental Computations, *ACM Transactions on Programming Languages and Systems,* 13(2):181–210.

Yoshikazu T., K. Iwasawa, Y. Umetani and S. Gotou. 1990. Compiling Techniques for First-Order Linear Recurrences on a Vector Computer, *Transactions on Programming Languages and Systems,* 4(1).

Zadeck, F. K. 1984. *Incremental Data Flow Analysis in a Structured Program Editor,* Proceedings of the ACM SIGPLAN Symposium on Compiler Construction, 132–143.

Ziegler, S. F. 1990. *Production Quality Portability,* SIGPLAN '90 Advanced Topics Tutorial, White Plains, New York.

EXERCISES

1. Discuss storage issues for *records, sets,* and *enumerated types* using the discussion of arrays in Section 11.3.13 as a model.

2. Give two criteria necessary for static storage allocation. Explain why this prohibits both recursion and nesting.

3. Using the grammar for arrays in Section 11.3.13, devise semantic functions to accompany each production. Illustrate it with the array reference in Example 6.

4. If the grammar for array references in Section 11.3.13 is rewritten so that the name of the array is at the bottom of the tree, the attributes can be evaluated in one pass up the tree. Rewrite the grammar (and the semantic functions) using the array reference in Example 6.

5. Symbol Tables: The language issues discussed in Section 11.3 apply to symbol table structures as well as to run-time systems. Discuss appropriate symbol table structures for each of the following: (i) static variables, (ii) semi-static variables, (iii) semi-dynamic variables, (iv) dynamic variables. What is the influence of recursion and block structure?

6–8. Consider the following nesting structure:

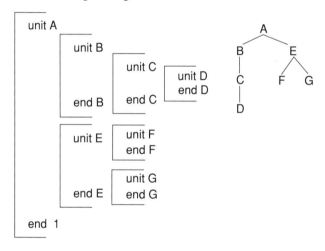

6. Consider the graph of stacks over time and the point marked with the asterisks, ***:

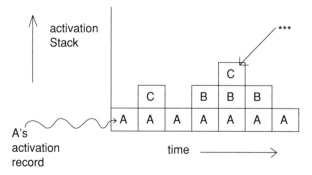

How is a variable X accessed if it is used in C, but defined in A?

7. Suppose A calls E calls F calls G calls F calls G calls F. Show the stack of activation records at this point including return pointers to code and static and dynamic links.

8. Displays: An alternative to static chains for implementing block structure is a data structure called a *display*. A display is an array of pointers to activation records along the chain. The display is updated so that *Display*[*i*] points to the correct activation record for a procedure at nesting level *i*. Show the sequence of display pointers for the sequence of procedure calls in Exercises 6 and 7. The display will contain the correct value if each procedure at nesting level *i* stores the old value (perhaps in the activation record) for *Display*[*i*] and restores it when the activation record is removed from the stack.

9. Comment on the following statement as it applies to the run-time system for languages that support recursion: "One doesn't *have* to use a stack. Local objects from previous activation records could exist forever."

10. Compaction: Garbage collection recovers unused storage. A technique called compaction moves the currently used storage so that it is consecutive, thus keeping memory from becoming too fragmented. Write a high-level procedure to perform compaction.

11. Analyze your favorite computer system—the machine, operating system and other system software. What would need to be done to port a language to this system? Answer for a specific language. If you are familiar with more than one system, discuss the issues in porting from each of the systems to the other.

Compiler Project
Run-Time Systems ***Optional***

Write a run-time system for the language of your project. You should allow for recursion, but not necessarily for nested procedures. If you choose this option, then you may wish to write an interpreter at code generation time instead of generating assembly language code. The interpreter uses the run-time system and the intermediate representation of a program to execute it. This option will have to be chosen if the system you are using does not have an assembler or if you do not wish to use it.

Run your compiler on a recursive algorithm such as Quicksort.

12

Compiling for
Special Architectures

12.0   Introduction

Early computers of the 1940's and 50's had small instruction sets which executed on a small number of also small (often 8-bit) registers. Hardware was expensive, and compiler techniques were just developing. Floating-point operations, often implemented in software, were slow.

The 1960's and 70's saw a decrease in the price of hardware and the introduction of designs which modeled high-level language constructs such as loop instructions and array indexing. Many of these constructs were implemented in microcode; for this reason machine instructions were themselves translated to lower-level sequences of (micro-)code. These machines, when compared with reduced instruction set computers (RISC's), are called CISC's—Complex Instruction Set Computers.

Much of the information in this chapter applies equally well to CISC machines. Separation of the RISC discussion from parallel architecture issues is also somewhat artificial since RISC architectures may also be parallel architectures. We have avoided discussing specific machines and processors and discuss only their features. The related reading (Section 12.5) refers to specific architectures (or a reference's bibliography does!).

One strong point exists for compiling for special architectures. This is that the hardware chip design and (optimizing) compiler design have often proceeded hand in hand. Rarely today is the compiler designer faced with a hardware design for which no consideration of how it is to be used has been made.

12.1   Compiling for RISC Machines

Interactions between programmers and hardware designers resulted in the hardware implementation of high-level language constructs. This led to large instruction sets and the proliferation of addressing modes. Research into the use of these complex instructions and addressing modes began to show that a small number of instructions and modes were used most frequently. For example, three of the DEC VAX™'s ten addressing modes account for 85% of the use; ten of the over 200 instructions on the IBM 370™ accounted for 67% of use [Muchnick, 1990].

Reduced Instruction Set Computers (RISC) are designed to reflect this simplicity. The return to smaller instruction sets and simpler addressing modes is not a return to the past, however. Random access memory is faster and cheaper. Registers and buses remain larger (generally 32 bits). Hardware design and implementation as well as compiler techniques are much better understood.

Nevertheless, RISC machines pose interesting problems for compiler designers, particularly in the areas of optimization and code generation. Because there are a larger number of registers, more program quantities can be kept in registers. Source level debugging of this highly optimized code has become a challenge.

12.1.1   RISC Machine Features

There is some controversy concerning what is or is not a RISC processor. The debate centers upon whether to classify a machine as RISC, as opposed to CISC, by architectural differences such as an abundance of registers or by performance measures such as performance of benchmark programs. In this section, we mention a number of architectural features commonly associated with RISC machines.

Small, Simpler Instruction Set and Few Addressing Modes

Small, simple and *few* are relative terms. Instruction set sizes are typically less than 150. Four or fewer addressing modes are common, although some processors have more.

Instruction set formats tend to be fixed in size, in contrast to variable length instruction formats of CISC machines. The number of these fixed-length formats is small, often on the order of two or three. This results in a faster (hard-wired) decoding.

Single-cycle operations allow the instructions to execute rapidly. *Load-Store* design dictates that only Load and Store instructions access memory. Ideally, these are the only instructions which take more than one machine cycle to execute.

Elimination of complex instructions eliminates the need for microcode.

Many Registers

Operations execute faster when the data is in a register. Thirty-two or more registers are common for RISC machines. Some have more. Hardware maintained sets of registers, called *register windows*, are organized in a circular queue, with a new set added to the tail of the queue and an older set removed from the head of the queue.

Levels of Memory

In addition to secondary memory, and a large number of registers, RISC processors include cache memory. Sometimes there is a separate cache memory for operations and operands. There may be separate buses to each cache.

Special-Purpose Architectures

RISC machines are often designed for a particular application or language or operating system. There are RISC machines for signal processing, symbolic processing, AI, image processing, scientific calculations, graphics processing, multiprocessing, and parallel processing. In addition, there are several general-purpose RISC machines on the market.

12.1.2   Compiler Issues in RISC Machines

Some of the issues that follow are also common to CISC machines and to recent languages such as Ada. They are mentioned here because compiler designers for RISC architectures have found them particularly important.

Pipelining

Pipelining traditionally has been the process of fetching instructions or data while another instruction is executing. It becomes increasingly important on RISC processors. Because all computations must take place in registers, and loads and stores access memory, it is important for the compiler to reorder code when it can so that the CPU is executing while a load or store is taking place. Since it is estimated that 1/3 of a program's executable instructions involve loads and stores, this is an especially important task. Pipelining has also been used to try to sustain an execution rate of more than one instruction/cycle [Smith et al., 1989a].

Register Usage

Because RISC computations take place in registers and are one cycle or less, but a load takes more than one cycle, a technique called *scoreboarding* has been developed. When an instruction is begun whose result will affect a register, that register is marked on a scoreboard. This mark is erased when the instruction concludes (and the register has its new data). Other instructions check the scoreboard, and if they need the results from that register, the CPU waits. A clever compiler can keep these CPU waiting periods to a minimum.

If all program quantities are kept in registers, a speed-up of as much as 1/3 can be expected from the program. A large number of registers facilitates this, but even these must be used effectively.

Because of the large number of registers, it is often possible to keep each operand in a register and store the result in yet another register, thus allowing both operands to remain in a register for a possible future use.

A technique called *value tracking* keeps a list of program quantities whose values are currently in registers. A set of ordered pairs (Value, Register) is maintained, and when the value is needed for another computation, it is fetched from the register.

Registers may be organized into a file of (possibly overlapping) register sets. When these sets are managed by the hardware, they are called *register windows*. Register windows allow for fast storing and restoring of information in procedure calls. These register windows are organized into a circular queue rather than the traditional stack which stores and restores for each call. A new procedure call (automatically) increments a pointer so that the outgoing parameter registers become the ingoing parameter registers for the new procedure. A return operation reverses this process.

Optimization and Code Generation Techniques

Since loads and stores may slow execution, it is important for the code generator to minimize them. Peephole optimization techniques can remove redundant loads or unnecessary stores.

A two-cycle instruction such as a branch has to compute an address. Execution cannot continue until after the address is computed. A technique known as *delayed branching* moves the branch instruction back one instruction so that the statement preceding the branch is executed at the same time that the address is being calculated. Another technique is to execute the instruction after a conditional branch at the same time as the address fetch (hoping that the branch doesn't take place).

Other standard optimizations, such as computing common subexpressions once, and good register allocation, such as that performed by coloring, can improve RISC programs by higher percentages. One performance estimate for a RISC compiler vs. the same compiler on a CISC machine found the improvement on the RISC machine to be about 50% with nowhere near that much improvement on the CISC machine.

Run-time checks can sometimes be eliminated by the compiler. Checking that a variable $X1$ in the expression $X1 := A + BB * 12$ is within its declared bounds of say $0 .. 255$, is not needed at run time if the compiler knows that A is declared as $0 .. 100$ and B is declared as $0 .. 10$. Of course, checks for A and B are still needed unless a similar dependence can also be found at compile time. On RISC machines, this sort of compiler simulation can cost as much as 20% in compile time, but may remove as many as 70% of the run-time checks.

Inlining is the replacement of a procedure call with the code of the called procedure. Even with register windowing, this can produce a program which runs faster at the expense of a (perhaps huge) increase in code space. Inlining is most productive when there are lots of calls to very short procedures.

Because the typical RISC architecture does not have microcode, the translated code is "bare-bones", exposing code sequences to optimizations which may have been hidden on CISC machines.

Debugger Interaction

Production-quality compilers produce code in the object file format of the machine. It is this structure to which the debugger refers. If there is a one-one correspondence between a source program construct and its place in the object file, then debugging is facilitated. In heavily optimized code, this may not be the case.

Debugging of optimized code is a challenge in any architecture—CISC or RISC. If a computation, say a loop invariant one, has been moved, and a programmer steps to that instruction point, the expected instruction is not there. Ideally, the debugger should try to figure out what the compiler has done and either undo it or inform the programmer. This may mean that the compiler should leave this information in the object file for the debugger.

Another problem arises from the register window situation. If a variable has been kept in a register during one procedure execution, and the programmer asks to see that variable's value when executing another procedure (and another register window), the debugger has to be informed that the variable is no longer in that register.

Debugging *inlined* code (see above) is also a difficult task. A bug in a procedure has now been reproduced as many times as the inlined procedure is called. Compilers, ideally, should leave information in the object module's symbol file, indicating that a piece of code had really only been written by the programmer once.

12.2   Compiling in a Parallel Processing Environment

Parallel processing which overlaps fetch and execute instructions at both the hardware level and the compiler level is not new. Instruction pipelining is actually an example of parallel processing.

12.2.1   Parallel Machine Features

RISC architectures are often parallel processing environments. Other parallel processing environments include multiple CPU's (multiprocessing) and multiple ALU's (array processors and supercomputers) and systems with enough back-up components to execute even if there is a hardware error (fault-tolerant computers).

Multiple processors which have their own memory and I/O ports (loosely coupled systems) have different compiler issues from those which have multiple CPU's, but share memory and I/O ports (tightly coupled systems).

12.2.2   Compiling in a Multiprocessing Environment

Preparing code to execute in more than one processor involves synchronization. Values which are needed in one processor may be computed in another. Changes in shared memory must be done carefully.

An interesting example of parallel execution in a multiprocessing environment is execution of the compiler itself. In some environments, the compiler is the major software process.

One technique for producing code for parallel processing environments is to take a compiler which produces code in a non-parallel processing environment and write a scheduler for the produced code to execute on parallel execution units. This can be done automatically, using the best developed techniques and heuristics, or in interactive mode with the (knowledgeable) programmer hand-tuning the automatically produced code.

12.2.3   Compiling for Array Processors and Supercomputers

Array processors (sometimes called vector machines) and supercomputers use parallelism to increase performance. Typically, these machines are used to perform high-precision arithmetic calculations on large arrays. In addition, they may need to operate in real time or close to real time.

Supercomputers are also used for general-purpose computing, while array processors are special-purpose (often peripheral) processors which operate solely on vectors.

Discovering data dependencies is one of the major issues for these architectures.

Data Dependencies

Data dependence checking is important for detecting possibilities for parallel scheduling of serial code. Strictly speaking, the problem is one of *concurrency*. For example, the following statements cannot be executed at the same time:

```
X := Y + 1
Z := X + 2
```

Since *X*'s value is needed to compute *Z*, the second statement depends on the first. The following statements could be executed in parallel:

```
X := Y + 1
Z := Y + 2
```

Parallelization, like optimization, has a potentially higher payoff in loops. The following loop can be changed to execute in parallel:

```
FOR I := 1 TO AHighNumber
  A[I] := A[I] + B[I]
ENDFOR
```

For two processors this could become:

```
FOR I := 1 TO AHighNumber BY 2
  A[I] := A[I] + B[I]
  A[I+1] := A[I + 1] + B[I + 1]
ENDFOR
```

This is called *loop unrolling*. Since each statement within the loop is affecting and using a separate element of the array, the two statements can be executed in parallel. There will be half as many test and branch instructions to execute since the loop is now counting by 2's.

Some machines have numerous processors. On a machine with 64 processors, the following

```
FOR I := 1 TO N * 64
  A[I] := A[I] + B[I]
ENDFOR
```

might become

```
FOR I := 0 TO N - 1 DO
  FOR J := 64 * I + 1 TO 64 * I + 64 DO
    A[J] := A[J] + B[J]
  ENDFOR
ENDFOR
```

The inner loop statement can now be executed simultaneously on all 64 processors.

The statement in the following loop contains a data dependency and cannot be effectively parallelized:

```
FOR I := 1 TO AHighNumber
  A[I] := A[I - 1] + B[I]
ENDFOR
```

Here, the value computed in one iteration of the loop is used in the next iteration so that the loop cannot be unrolled and processed in parallel.

Debugger Interaction

Producing information in the object module which the debugger can use is important since there may no longer be a one-one correspondence between the code produced by the programmer and that which is scheduled for parallel execution. If the technique of scheduling code after the compiler has produced it is used, then there isn't even a one-one correspondence between the code produced by the compiler and that being executed by the debugger. In this case, the scheduler should leave a trail for the debugger to follow.

12.2.4 Super-Scalar Processors

Processors capable of executing *more* than one instruction per cycle are termed *super-scalar processors*. Architecturally, they combine RISC features with parallel processing. To maintain an instruction rate of two instructions per cycle requires sophisticated branch prediction.

Much is known about achieving concurrency for scientific calculations, but for wider applications, non-vectorizable instruction concurrency is needed.

Algorithms for finding non-numerical instructions which can be executed in parallel in a general application or business application environment are needed.

12.3 Compiling in a Fault-Tolerant Environment

Previous sections of this chapter have described special architecture for increasing performance. There is also a growing need for systems that "produce correct results or actions even in the presence of faults or other anomalous or unexpected conditions" [Singh, 1990]. Fault-tolerant systems increase dependability through redundancy. Applications such as robotics, navigational systems and others require reliable systems. The purpose of a fault-tolerant system is to be able to execute an algorithm in the presence of hardware or software errors. Fault tolerance may be implemented in hardware with back-up devices or in software.

12.3.1 Fault-Tolerant Hardware Features

Fault-tolerant machines have a back-up for every critical part of the machine. This includes the CPU, I/O ports, buses, and the ALU.

12.3.2 Fault-Tolerant Software Features

Fault tolerance can be simulated in software. For example, Ancona et al. (1990) describes a number of software techniques. One example of such a technique is the sequence

```
ensure | x² - y | < tolerable
by x := SqrtA(y)
else x := SqrtB(y)
else error
```

Here, multiple versions of a function which computes a square root are provided, increasing the likelihood that the square root value returned satisfies some criterion.

Knowledgeable compilers which produce code for fault-tolerant systems should be aware of the redundancies in the architecture. Much research is needed to make this a reality.

12.4 Summary

Although there is disagreement on exactly what qualifies as a RISC machine, char-
acterizations include [Tabak, 1986] (1) as small an instruction set as possible, (2) as
small a set of addressing modes as possible, (3) as small a number of instruction formats as possible, (4) single-cycle execution of as many instructions as possible, (5)
memory access by load-store instructions only, (6) number of user general-purpose
registers as large as possible, (7) no microcode, (8) high-level language support.

The type of benchmark program used to test a computer often affects the results.
For example, programs such as Quicksort or Towers of Hanoi contain lots of recursive subprogram calls. It is not surprising, therefore, that these programs show a sub-
stantial improvement when executed on RISC machines with register windowing to
efficiently handle the overhead of calls and returns.

Programming for parallel environments involves two approaches: (1) learning
how to program for concurrency and using languages which facilitate this and (2)
scheduling of already-written sequential code for parallel processing.

Throughout this chapter the topic of *parallelism* is discussed. RISC architectures
are often parallel. Fault tolerance is often implemented in the presence of parallelism. Parallelism makes programs run faster. Parallelism makes programs run safer.
The need for both fast and safe executions is a challenge.

New architectures continue to evolve. Their effective use requires constant study
of the applications for which they are intended and compiler techniques which will
exploit the new architecture.

12.5 Related Reading

Albert, E., K. Knobe, J. Lukas, and G. Steele Jr. 1988. Compiling Fortran 8x Array Features
for the Connection Machine Computer System, *SIGPLAN Notices,* 23(9):42–56.
> *Describes some optimizations for minimizing transfers and context-switching between the
> Connection machine and a VAX as well as some standard optimizations.*

Allen, F., B. Rosen, and F. K. Zadeck. 1990. *Optimization in Compilers*, ACM Press-Addison
Wesley.

Allen, J. and K. Kennedy. 1987. Automatic Translation of Fortran to Vector Form, *ACM
Transactions on Programming Languages and Systems,* 4:491–542.

Ancona, M., G. Dodero, V. Giant, A. Clement and E. B. Fernandez. 1990. A System Architecture for Fault Tolerance in Concurrent Software, *IEEE Computer,* 23(10).
> *A recovery component, separate from the application program, coordinates the applica-
> tion program's execution.*

Barry, R. 1988. An Attribute Grammar for Building Intraprocedural Data Dependence Graphs,
Master's thesis, Worcester MA: Worcester Polytechnic Institute.

Burke, M. and R. Cytron. 1986. *Interprocedural Dependence Analysis, and Parallelization*,
Proceedings of ACM SIGPLAN Symposium on Compiler Construction, 162–175.

Callahan, D. and K. Kennedy. 1988. Compiling Programs for Distributed-Memory Multipro-
cessors, *The Journal of Supercomputing,* 2:151–169.

Chow, F. and J. Hennessy. 1990. The Priority-Based Coloring Approach to Register Allocation. *ACM Transactions on Programming Languages and Systems,* 12(4):501–536.

Chow, F., M. Himelstein, E. Killian, and L. Weber. 1986. *Engineering a RISC Compiler System*, Proc. COMPCON s'86, 132–137.

Cohen, P. E. 1988. An Abundance of Registers, *SIGPLAN Notices*, 23(6):24–34.
Discusses register allocation and assignment in the environment of many (32) registers.

Colwell, R. P., C. Y. Hitchcock III, E. D. Jensen, H. M. Brinkley Sprint, and C. Kollar. 1985. Computers, Complexity and Controversy, *IEEE Computer*, Sept.:8–19.
One of the first articles to propose a working definition of a RISC machine.

Coutant, D., C. Hammond, and J. Kelly. 1986. *Compilers for the New Generation of Hewlett-Packard Computers*, Proc. COMPCON s'86, 48–61.

Cristian, F. 1991. Understanding Fault-Tolerant Distributed Systems, *CACM*, 34(2):57–78.

Falk, H. 1988. 88000 Designed for Use with Optimizing Compilers, *Computer Design*, May:30–32.
Describes how the M88000 designers considered the actions of optimizing compilers in the design of the 88000.

Falk, H. 1988. Optimizing Compilers Address Debugging and User Control Constraints, *Computer Design*, July:48–56.
The problem of optimized code debugging is addressed in the context of new technologies and increased user insistence on some control of the optimization process.

Fortes, J. A. B. and D. I. Moldovan. 1985. Parallel Detection and Transformation Techniques Useful for VLSI Algorithms, *Journal of Parallel and Distributed Computing*, 2(3):277–301.

Gajski, D. D., D. A. Padua, D. J. Kuck and R. H. Kuhn. 1982. A Second Opinion on Data Flow Machines and Languages, *IEEE Computer*, 15(2).

Gimarc, C. E. and V. M. Milutinovic. *A Survey of RISC Processors and Computers of the Mid-1980's.*
Surveys a number of RISC machines and emphasizes the importance of optimizing compilers for them.

Gupta, R. and M. L. Soffa. 1989. Compilation Techniques for a Reconfigurable LIW Architecture, *Journal of Super Computing*, 3(4).

Hennessy, J. L. and D. A. Patterson. 1990. *Computer Architecture: A Quantitative Approach*, San Mateo, CA: Morgan Kaufmann.

Insinga, A. and K. A. Lemone. 1987. *Parsing in a Multiprocessor Environment*, Proceedings of the 1987 ACM Computer Science Conference.

Hseush, W. and G. Kaiser. 1990. Modeling Concurrency in Parallel Debugging, *SIGPLAN Notices*, 25(7):11–19.

Krick, R. and A. Dallas. 1991. The Evolution of Instruction Sequencing, *Computer*, 24(4):5–15.

Krishnamurthy, S. M. 1990. A Brief Survey of Papers on Scheduling for Pipelined Processors, *SIGPLAN Notices*, 25(7).
Reviews a number of people's work in optimization for pipelining.

Lam, M. 1988. *Compiler Optimizations for Asynchronous Systolic Array Programs*, Proceedings 15th POPL Conference.

Lengauer, C. 1990. *Code Generation for a Systolic Computer*, 20(3).

Midkiff, S. D., and D. A. Padua. 1987. Compiler Algorithms for Synchronization, *IEEE Transactions on Computers*, 36(12).

Muchnick, S. S. *Compiling for RISC-Based Systems*, SIGPLAN '90 Advanced Topics Tutorial.
Describes features of some commercial RISC architectures.

Nelson, V. P. 1990. Fault-Tolerant Computing: Fundamental Concepts, *IEEE Computer*, 23(7):15–17.
Describes hardware for fault-tolerant systems.

Oldehoeft, R. R. and D. C. Cann. 1988. Applicative Parallelism on a Shared-Memory Multiprocessor, *IEEE Software*, 5(1).

Oyang, Y. 1991. Exploiting Multi-way Branching to Boost Superscalar Processor Performance, *SIGPLAN Notices*, 26(3):68–78.

Padua, D. A. and M. J. Wolfe. 1986. Advanced Compiler Optimizations for Supercomputers, *CACM*, 29:1184–1201.
Describes techniques for detection of parallelism in vectorizing compilers.

Patterson, D. A. 1985. Reduced Instruction Set Computers, *CACM*, 28(1):8–21.

Ruighaver, A. B. and T. T. E. Yeo. 1990. Language Support for a Semi-dataflow Parallel Programming Environment, *SIGPLAN Notices*, 25(9).
Describes features of a prototype parallel programming language which expects that the machine dependent optimizations take care of efficient execution on both sequential and parallel architectures.

Sacks, R. 1989. Detecting Interprocedural Parallelism During Semantic Analysis, Master's thesis, Worcester, MA: Worcester Polytechnic Institute.
Sequential programs are analyzed to find the procedures which may be processed in parallel.

Schell, R. M. 1979. Methods for Constructing Parallel Compilers for Use in a Multiprocessor Environment, Ph.D. dissertation, Univ. of Illinois, Urbana.
Adds two more actions—cancel and continue—to the standard LR-parsing actions. Parallel processing of other compiler phases also discussed.

Singh, A. D. and S. Murugesan. 1990. Fault-Tolerant Systems, *IEEE Computer*, 23(7):15–17.
An introduction to a special edition on fault-tolerant systems.

Smith, M. D., M. Johnson, and M. Horowitz. 1989a. *Limits on Multiple Instruction Issue*, Proceedings of the 3rd International Conference on Architectural Support for Programming Languages and Operating Systems, Boston, 290–302.
Discusses techniques and barriers for maintaining an instruction execution rate of two cycles per second.

Smith, M. D., M. Johnson, and M. Horowitz. 1989b. *Boosting Beyond Static Scheduling in a Superscalar Processor*, Proceedings of the 3rd International Conference on Architectural Support for Programming Languages and Operating Systems, Boston, 344–354.
Presents a technique called boosting which executes instructions across basic block boundaries, to improve concurrency in non-numerical applications.

Stallings, W. 1990. *Reduced Instruction Set Computers*, 2nd ed., Los Alamitos, CA: IEEE Computer. Soc. Press.

Tabak, D. 1986. Which System Is a RISC in the Open Channel, *IEEE Computer,* October:85–86.

Treleaven, P. C. and O. G. Lima. 1984. Future Computers: Logic, Data Flow, Control Flow, *IEEE Computer,* 17(3).

Tseng, P. S. 1990. *Compiling Programs for a Linear Systolic Array*, Proceedings of the ACM SIGPLAN '90 Conference on Programming Language Design and Implementation, White Plains, NY, 311–321.

Veen, A. H. 1986. *The Misconstrued Semicolon: Reconciling Imperative Languages, and Dataflow Machines*, Amsterdam: Centrum voor Wiskunde en Informatica.

Wall, D. 1987. *Register Windows vs. Register Allocation*, DEC Western Res. Lab Research Report 87/5, Dec.

Williams, T. 1990. Optimizing Compilers Struggle to Meet the Challenge of Silicon, *Computer Design,* April:67–78.
Emphasizes that compiler designers and chip designers must work together to produce optimized code that can be debugged.

Wirth, N. 1987. *Hardware Architectures for Programming Languages and Programming Languages for Hardware Architectures*, Keynote address in Proceedings of 2nd International Conference on Architectural Support for Programming Languages and Operating Systems, 2–8.
Emphasizes that compilers can aid in the efficiency of implementing parallelism, but that hardware as well as the compiler bears a responsibility for enforcing correctness.

Wolfe, M. and U. Banerjee. 1987. Data Dependence and Its Application to Parallel Processing, *International Journal of Parallel Programming,* 16(2):137–178.

EXERCISES

1. Using the related reading as a starting point, research the number of instructions, addressing modes, etc. of RISC machines. Distinguish between prototype machines and commercially available systems.

2. What phases and techniques in a compiler aid in the process of pipelining?

3. Can the following statements be executed in parallel. Why or why not?

    (a) X := B + 1
       B := Y + 2
    (b) X := 2
       Y := X + 1
       X := 3

4. A program is *vectorizable* if it can be executed correctly on a set of tightly coupled (synchronized) processors; a program is *concurrentizable* if it can be executed correctly on a set of loosely coupled (asynchronous) processors.

Which of these descriptions is applicable to each of these FORTRAN code segments?*

(a)   DO 10 I = 1,100
     10 A(I) = A(I) + B(I) * C(I)
(b)   DO 10 I = 2,100
     10 A(I) = A(I - 1) + B(I) * C(I)
(c)   DO 10 I = 1,99
     10 A(I) = A(I + 1) + B(I) * C(I)

* From GBC/ACM *Real Times*, Sept. 1991.

Appendix A

Answers to Selected Exercises

Chapter 1

1. (e) Good field service support, perhaps even training in using the tool
   (f) Help-line number, (g) ...

2. (a) Using regular expressions as the input, and assuming a function *Output* which prints out tokens as an ordered pair

```
Letter = A | a | B | b | ... Z | z
Digit  = 0 | 1 | 2 ... | 9
Ident  = Letter | Letter Digit    {Output "Ident"}
Assign = ":="                     {Output ":="}
Punct  = ";"                      {Output ";"}
```

   (b) (Ident, "Max") (Assign, "=") (Ident, "A") (Punct, ";") (Ident, "This") (Assign, ":=") (Ident, "That") (Punct, ";")

   (c) (Lots of answers here, but be sure your grammar generates more than one assignment statement)

```
Program                → SequenceOfStatements
SequenceOfStatements   → Statement SequenceOfStatements
                         | Statement
Statement              → Assign
Assign                 → Ident ":=" Ident ";"
```

   (d)

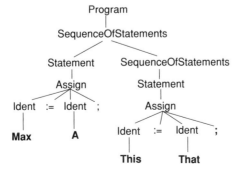

283

7. Identifier = Letter | Letter (Letter | Digit | $ | _)⁺ or Identifier = Letter
   (Letter | Digit | $ | _)*

8 .

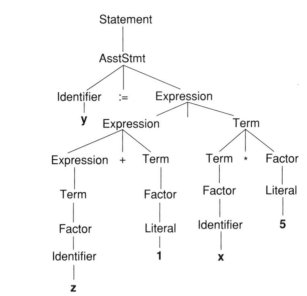

9. More tokens increases the work for the front-end while decreasing the work in
   the back-end (code generator).

Chapter 3

1. Hard to tell definition from limited examples, but the following will allow all
   the examples. Other answers possible.
   (a) `Digit = 0 | 1 | 2 | ... | 9`
       `Sign = + | -`
       `Real = Digit⁺.(Digit[E Sign Digit⁺])`⁺ with usual definition
       of digit
   (b) `Ident = $ (Letter | Digit | $)`* `$` with usual definition of let-
       ters and digits

3.
State / Input	[a ... z]	[A ... Z]	[0 ... 9]	Other
0	1	1	2	...
1	1	1	1	(Retract)
				(Return Id) 0

6.

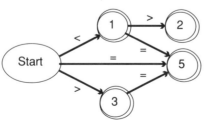

Chapter 4

6. Given: S → X X
            X → **x** X
            X → **y**

    (a) LL(1): FIRST (**x** X) ∩ FIRST (**y**) = φ
    (b) Parse table:

	x	**y**
S	S → X X	S → X X
X	X → **x** X	X → **y**

   (c) Parsing **x y x y**:

Stack (Top on Right)	Input	Production
$ S	**x y x y** $	S → X X
$ X X	**x y x y** $	X → **x** X
$ X X **x**	**x y x y** $	(Match)
$ X X	**y x y** $	X → **y**
$ X **y**	**y x y** $	(Match)
$ X	**x y** $	X → **x** X
$ X **x**	**x y** $	(Match)
$ X	**y** $	X → **y**
$ **y**	**y** $	(Match)
$	$	(Accept)

7. FIRST (E) = { **(**, **Id**} because
   (: E → T → F → **(**E)
   Id : E → T → F → **Id**

   FOLLOW (T) = {**+**,**)**} because
   + : E → T E' → T **+** T E'
) : E → T E' → F T' E' → **(**E) T' E' → **(**T E'**)** T' E'
        → **(**T**)** . . .

9. (a) Lots of choices for 2 parse trees for same string
    (b) An ambiguous grammar cannot be LL(1):

    Consider derivation S ⇒⃰ α A β ⇒¹ α γ₁ β ⇒⃰ ω

                        ⇒⃰ α A β ⇒² α γ₂ β ⇒⃰ ω

    where Derivation 1 ≠ Derivation 2 (Such a derivation exists because grammar is ambiguous).
    Then, FIRST (γ₁) ∩ FIRST (γ₂) ≠ ø

11.
    E → E + T ⇒⃰ **Id** + T

    E → E - T ⇒⃰ **Id** - T

12. (a) Not LL(1):   For S' → **e** S and S' → ε,
                            FIRST(**e** S) ∩ FOLLOW(S') = {**e**} ≠ ϕ

   (b) Table (note multiple entry at Table[S',**e**]):

	i	**a**	**e**	**c**
S	S → **i** EtS S'	S → **a**		
S'			S' → **e** S	
			S' → ε	
E				E → **c**

   (c)

Stack	Input	Production
(Top on right)		
$ S	i c t i c t a e a $	S → **i** E **t** S S'
$ S' S **t** E **i**	i c t i c t a e a $	Match
$ S' S **t** E	c t i c t a e a $	E → **c**
$ S' S **t** c	c t i c t a e a $	Match
$ S' S **t**	t i c t a e a $	Match
$ S' S	i c t a e a $	S → **i** E **t** S S'
$ S' S' S **t** E **i**	i c t a e a $	Match
$ S' S' S **t** E	c t a e a $	E → **c**
$ S' S' S **t** c	c t a e a $	Match
$ S' S' S **t**	t a e a $	Match
$ S' S' S	a e a $	S → **a**
$ S' S' **a**	a e a $	Match
$ S'S'	a e $	S' → **e** S (choice 1)
$ S' S **e**	e a $	Match
$ S' S	a $	S → **a**
$ S' **a**	a $	Match
$ S'	$	S' → ε
$	$	**Accept**

Chapter 5

2. Grammar: 0. S' → S
            1. S → S A
            2. S → A
            3. **A** → **Id** := E ;
            4. E → E + T
            (etc.)

New beginning states:

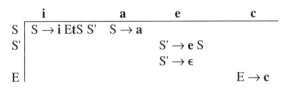

State 0	State 1	State 2	State 3
S' → • S	S' → S •	S'→ **A** •	A → **Id** • := E ;
S → • S **A**	S → S • **A**		
S → • **A**	A → • **Id** := E ;		
A → • **Id** := E ;			

State 4	State 5	State 6	State 8

State 4
S → S **A** •

State 5
A → **Id** := • E ;
E → • E **+** T
E → • T
T → • T * F
T → • F
F → • (E)
F → • **Id**

State 6
A → **Id** := E • ;
E → E • **+** T

State 7
E → T •
T → T • * F

State 8
T → F •

State 9
F → (• E)
E → • E **+** T
E → • T
T → • T * F
T → • F
F → • (E)
F → • **Id**

State 10
F → **Id** •

State 11
A → **Id** := E ; •

State 12
E → E **+** • T

State 13
T → T * • F

State 14
F → (E •)
E → E • **+** T

State 15
E → T •
T → T • * F

State 16
E → E **+** T •

State 17
T→ T * F •

State 18
F → (E) •

3. (a) 0. S' → S
   1. S → Adj**s Noun Verb Adjs** •
   2. Adjs → **Adj** , Adjs
   3. Adjs → **And Adj**
   4. Adjs → **ϵ**

(b)
State 0
S' → • S
S → • Adjs **Noun Verb Adjs** .
Adjs → • **Adj** , Adjs
Adjs → • **And Adj**
Adjs → • **ϵ**

State 1
S' → S •

State 2
S → Adjs • **Noun Verb Adjs** .

State 3
Adjs → **Adj**• , Adjs

State 4
Adjs → **And** • **Adj**

State 5
S → Adjs **Noun** • **Verb Adjs** .

State 6
S → Adjs **Noun Verb** • **Adjs** .
Adjs → • **Adj** , Adjs
Adjs → • **And Adj**
Adjs → • **ϵ**

State 7
S → Adjs **Noun Verb Adjs** • .

State 8
S → Adjs **Noun Verb Adjs** . •

State 9
Adjs → **And Adj** •

State 10
Adjs → **Adj** , • Adjs
Adjs → • **Adj** , Adjs
Adjs → • **And Adj**
Adjs → • **ϵ**

State 11
Adjs → **Adj** , Adjs •

	A C T I O N S							**G O T O**	
State	Verb	Noun	Adj	.	,	AND	$	S	Adjs
0		R4	S3			S4		1	2
1							Acc.		
2		S5							
3					S10				
4			S9						
5	S6								
6			S3	R4		S4		7	
7					S8				
8							R1		
9		R3		R3					
10		R4	S3	R4		S4		11	
11		R2		R2					

Parsing the string

Bad, Muscular, and wicked Dudes are mean, nasty, and ugly.

that is,

Adj, Adj, AND Adj Noun Verb Adj, Adj, AND Adj.

Stack	**Input**	**Action**
$S0	Adj, Adj, AND Adj Noun Verb Adj, Adj, AND Adj. $	S3
$S0 Adj 3,	Adj, AND Adj Noun Verb Adj, Adj, AND Adj. $	S10
etc.		

(Note that lots of stuff gets pushed onto the stack before a reduction is made)

6. 0. S" → S (augmented production)
   1. S → i E t S S'
   2. S → a
   3. S' → e S
   4. S' → ε
   5. E → c

LR(0) States

State 0	**State 1**	**State 2**
S" → • S	S" → • S	S → i • E t S S'
S → • i E t S S'	(accept state)	E → • b
S → • a		

State 3	**State 4**	**State 5**
S → i E • t S S'	S → a •	E → b •
	(FOLLOW(S) = {e, $})	(FOLLOW(E) = {t})

State 6	**State 7**	**State 8**
S → i E t • S S'	S → i E t S • S'	S → i E t S S' •
S → • a	S' → • e S	(FOLLOW(S) = {e,$})
S → • i E t S S'	S' → • epsilon	(FOLLOW(S) = {e,$})

State 9

S' → e • S

S →• **i** E **t** S S'

S → • a

State 10

S'→ e S •

(FOLLOW(S') = {$})

(b) Parsing table

State	|	i	t	e	a	b	$	||	S	E	S'
				A C T I O N						**G O T O**	
0		S2			S4				1		
1							Acc.				
2						S5				3	
3			S6								
4				R2							
5			R5								
6		S2			S4				7		
7				S9			R4				8
8				R1			R1				
9		S2			S4				10		
10							R3				

Since there are no shift/reduce conflicts, grammar is SLR(1).

(c) Parsing *IF b THEN IF b THEN a ELSE a*

Stack	Input	Action
0	i b t i b t a e a $	S2
0i2	b t i b t a e a $	S5
0i2b5	t i b t a e a $	R5
0i2E3	t i b t a e a $	S6
0i2E3t6	i b t a e a $	S2
0i2E3t6i2	b t a e a $	S5
0i2E3t6i2b5	t a e a $	R5
0i2E3t6i2E3	t a e a $	S6
0i2E3t6i2E3t6	a e a $	S4
0i2E3t6i2E3t6a4	e a $	R2
0i2E3t6i2E3t6S7	e a $	S9
0i2E3t6i2E3t6S7e9a4	$	R2
0i2E3t6i2E3t6S7e9S10	$	R3
0i2E3t6i2E3t6S7S'8	$	R1
0i2E3t6S7	$	R4
0i2E3t6S7S'8	$	R1
0S1	$	Accept

Chapter 6

1. (b)

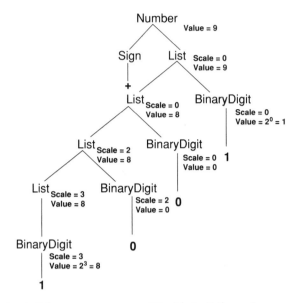

5. (a)

```
List → Id                          (i)  List.Ndim = 0
List → Id [ EList ]                (i)  List.Dims = Fetch(SymbolTable)
                                   (ii) EList.Dims = List.Dims

EList → Id
EList₀→ EList₁ , Id                (i)  EList₁.Dims = EList₀.Dims
```

An alternative is to use 2 attributes, 1 of which is the subscript of the other. Thus, d_{NDim} will use the fetched value of d_1, d_2, and d_3 (for a three-dimensional array) and assume that *NDim* is fetched at the same time as d_1, d_2, and d_3.

```
List → Id                          (i)  List.Ndim = 0
List → Id [ EList ]                (i)  List.NDim = Fetch(SymbolTable)
                                   (ii) FOR I := 1 TO NDim {gets d₁,
                                             d₂, and d₃} EList.dᵢ = List.dᵢ
                                                     = Fetch(SymbolTable)
                                        ENDFOR


EList → Id
EList₀→ EList₁ , Id                (i)  EList₁.NDim = EList₀.NDim - 1
                                   (ii) EList₁.d_{NDim} = List₀.d_{NDim}
```

Adding synthesized attribute *Offset* and *CheckDim:*

```
List → Id                          (i)  List.Ndim = 0
                                   (ii) List.CheckDim = 0
```

List → **Id** [EList]	(i) List.*NDim* = **Fetch**(SymbolTable)
	(ii) FOR I := 1 TO *NDim* {gets d_1, d_2, and d_3} EList.d_I = List.d_I = **Fetch**(Symbol Table) ENDFOR
	(iii) List.*CheckDim* = EList.*CheckDim*
	(iv) List.*Offset* = EList.*Offset*
EList → **Id**	(i) EList.*CheckDim* = 1
	(ii) EList.*Offset* = **LexVal**(Id) - 1
$\text{EList}_0 \rightarrow \text{EList}_1$, **Id**	(i) $\text{EList}_1.NDim = \text{EList}_0.NDim - 1$
	(ii) $\text{EList}_1.d_{NDim} = \text{List}_0.d_{NDim}$
	(iii) $\text{EList}_0.CheckDim = \text{EList}_1.CheckDim + 1$
	(iv) $\text{EList}_0.Offset = \text{EList}_1.Offset * \text{EList}_1.d_{NDim}$ + **LexVal**(Id) - 1

13. (a)

$E_0 \rightarrow E_1 + T$	$E_0.Value = E_1.Value + T.Value$
$E \rightarrow T$	$E_0.Value = T.Value$
$T_0 \rightarrow T_1 * F$	$T_0.Value = T_1.Value + F.Value$
$T \rightarrow F$	$T.Value = F Value$
F → (E)	$F.Value = E.Value$
F → **Const**	F.*Value* = **LexVal**(Const)

(b)

$E \rightarrow TE'$	$E.Value = T.Value + E'.Value$
$E_0 \rightarrow + TE_1'$	$E_0.Value = T.Value + E'_1.Value$
$E' \rightarrow \epsilon$	$E'.Value = 0$
$T \rightarrow F\ T'$	$T.Value = F.Value + T'.Value$
$T_0' \rightarrow *\ \mathbf{FT_1}'$	$T'_0.Value = F.Value + T'_1.Value$
$T' \rightarrow \epsilon$	$T'.Value = 1$
F → (E)	$F.Value = E.Value$
F → **Const**	F.*Value* = **LexVal**(Const)

14. (a) It is L-attributed
    (b) It is not LL(1)
    (c) It is S-attributed
    (d) It is LR(1)
    (Proofs are left to the reader. It should be easier knowing the answers.)

Chapter 7

2. (a) Dominators: Dom(S) = {S}, DOM(1) = {S,1}, DOM(2) = {S,1,2,8}, DOM(3) = {S,1,2,3,6,8}, Dom(4) = {S,1,2,3,4,6,8}, DOM(5) = {S,1,2,3,5,6,8}, DOM(6) = {S,1,2,6,8}, DOM(7) = {S,1,2,6,7,8}, DOM(8) = {S,1,8}
   (b) Back edges: B5 → B6, B7 → B8
   (c) Natural loops: {B3, B4, B5, B6}, {B2, B3, B4, B5, B6, B7, B8}

3. (a)

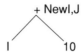

+ NewI,J

| 10

(Nodes can be created for the ":="'s or understood by the labeling)

(b)

Node		Left Child	Right Child
1.	I		
2.	10		
3.	+	(1)	(2)
4.	:=	NewI	(3)
5.	:=	J	(3)

5. (a, b)

```
            I := 1                    << Block 1
            GOTO ITest
    ILoop:  J := 1                    << Block 2
            GOTO JTest
    JLoop:  T1 := I * J               << Block 3
            T2 := 4 * T1
            Z[T2] := 0
            K := 1
            GOTO KTest
    KLoop:  T3 := I * J               << Block 4
            T4 := 4 * T3              ; [I,J]
            T5 := I * K
            T6 := 4 * T5              ; [I,K]
            T7 := K * J
            T8 := 4 * T7              ; [K,J]
            T9 := X[T6]
            T10 := Y[T8]
            T11:= Z[T4]
            T12 := T9 * T10           ; X[I,K] * Y[K,J]
            T13 := T12 + T11; + Z[I,J]
            Z[T4] := T13              ; Z[I,J] := X[I,K] * Y[K,J] + Z[I,J] K :=
                                       K + 1
    KTest:  IF K ≤ M GOTO KLoop       << Block 5
            J := J + 1                << Block 6
    JTest:  IF J ≤ N GOTO JLoop       << Block 7
            I := I + 1                << Block 8
    ITest:  IF I ≤ L GOTO ILoop       << Block 9
```

(c)

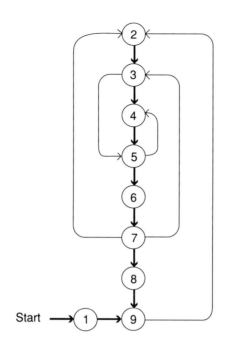

(d) (A) Depth-first order

```
    1 9 2 7 8 7 3 5 6 54 5 3 7 2 9 1
DFO: 1 9 2 7 3 5 4 6 8
```

(e) ```
Dom(1) = {1}
Dom(2) = {1,2,9}
Dom(3) = {1,2,3,7,9}
Dom(4) = {1,2,3,4,5,7,9}
Dom(5) = {1,2,3,5,7,9}
Dom(6) = {1,2,3,5,6,7,9}
Dom(7) = {1,2,7,9}
Dom(8) = {1,2,7,8,9}
Dom(9) = {1,9}
```

(f) 3 backedges: $4 \rightarrow 5$, $6 \rightarrow 7$, $8 \rightarrow 9$

(g) Natural loops: {4, 5}, {3, 4, 5, 6, 7}, {2, 3, 4, 5, 6, 7, 8, 9}
```

Chapter 8

1.

(a)

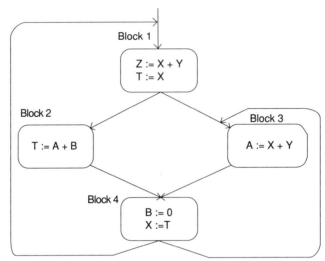

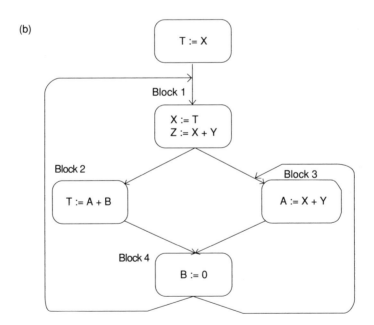

(b)

(This was really an exercise in understanding definitions. Compilers have little reason to change variables this way.)

7. It is circular; the value of the attribute following a GOTO is not necessarily in terms of attributes within the scope of a production.

9. **Pass 2:**

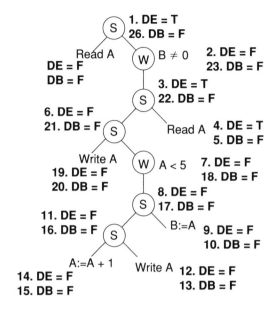

Pass 3: No changes

Chapter 9

1. (a) A := 4 * I + 4 * I
   or A := 2 * I + 2 * I + 2 * I + 2 * I
   or A := I + I + I + I + I + I + I + I
   (b) A := A * A

5. Because it is possible to enter and leave the loop without executing it.

8. Yes.

Chapter 12

4. Program (a) is both vectorizable and concurrentizable, since each A(I) is calculated independently. Program (c) is vectorizable, but not concurrentizable (the "old" value of A(I + 1) must be used to calculate A(I)), and progam (b) is neither. Timing restrictions may apply on actual vector processors.

Appendix B

Compiler Project SubAda

This project is easier than the one described in the text. Although the syntax is for a subset of Ada, it could easily be changed to a subset of most algorithmic languages.

Part I

Lexical Analysis

This project may be done following Chapter 3. Students often report times of 20–25 hours.

Consider the tokens (bolded) in the following subset of Ada:

Program	→	**begin** SequenceOfStatements **end ;**
SequenceOfStatements	→	Statement {Statement}
Statement	→	SimpleStatement | CompoundStatement
SimpleStatement	→	AssignmentStatement
AssignmentStatement	→	Name **:=** Expression **;**
Name	→	SimpleName
SimpleName	→	Identifier
Expression	→	Relation
Relation	→	SimpleExpression
SimpleExpression	→	Term {AddingOperator Term}
Term	→	Factor {MultiplyingOperator Factor}
Factor	→	Primary
Primary	→	Name | NumericLiteral | (Expression)
AddingOperator	→	**+** | **-**
MultiplyingOperator	→	***** | **/** | **mod** | **rem**
NumericLiteral	→	DecimalLiteral
DecimalLiteral	→	**Integer**
CompoundStatement	→	IfStatement | LoopStatement
IfStatement	→	**if** condition **then** SequenceOfStatements {**elsif** condition **then** SequenceOfStatements [**else** SequenceOfStatements] **end if ;**
LoopStatement	→	[iteration_scheme] **loop** SequenceOfStatements **end loop ;**

```
IterationScheme          → while condition
Condition                → Expression
Expression               → Relation {and Relation}
                           | Relation {or Relation}
                           | Relation {xor relation}
Relation                 → SimpleExpression [RelationalOperator
                           SimpleExpression]
RelationalOperator       → = | /= | < | <= | > | >=
```

Write regular expressions and transition diagrams for the tokens in the above grammar. Then:

Option 1 (Easier)   Using a compiler tool such as LEX, code the regular expressions for the tokens above and generate a lexical analyzer.

Option 2 (Easier)   Make the necessary changes to a given lexical analyzer (many tools include one) to find the tokens.

Option 3 (Much, much harder)   Using the methods of this chapter and the algorithms from Exercises 2 to 9, generate a lexical analyzer.

Run your lexical analyzer on the following input:

(a) ```
    begin
        a := b3 ;
        xyz := a + b + c
                      - p / q ;
        a := xyz * (p + q);
        p := a - xyz - p ;
    end;
```

(b) ```
    begin
        if i > j then
        i := i + j ;
        elsif i < j then
        i := 1 ;
        end if ;
    end;
```

(c) ```
    begin
        while (i < j) and (j < k) loop
        k := k + 1 ;
        while (i = j) loop
         i := i + 2 ;
        end loop;
        end loop;
    end;
```

(d) A program of your choice.

The output should consist of a list of tokens for each program. Each token in the list should include the characters in the token and its class.
```

Part II
Parser Generation

This project may be done after covering the material in Chapters 4 and 5. Students report times of 10–15 hours for this part of the project.

Consider the grammar for the subset of Ada in Part I.

Option 1 (Easier) Using a parser generator such as YACC, code the productions into the metalanguage of the tool and create a parser.

Option 2 (Harder) Following the description in Section 4.4, write a recursive descent parser.

Option 3 (Still harder) Generate a top-down parser for the grammar above.

Run your parser on the same input as in Chapter 1. Output should print the non-terminal on the left-hand side of the production whenever it is expanded (for top-down) or whenever it is reduced to (for bottom-up). A partial parse tree should be hand-drawn for each example (partial because it would take too much time and space to draw the entire tree for each example).

Part III
Error Handling (Optional)

Error handling involves four tasks:

(i) Error Creation This is not a problem (there are more incorrect programs than correct ones in the world), although some language designs make it easier for the programmer to make errors. Ada is well-designed in this respect, e.g., comments do not go over line boundaries, a common error source.

(ii) Error Detection Early detection finds the error, and as discussed in Section 5.3.1, both LL and LR parsers find the error as soon as it is pushed onto the stack.

(iii) Error Reporting Good error messages are important. The offending token should be named, perhaps by pointing to it in the source program, and an indication given as to why it is wrong.

(iv) Error Correction This is actually a misnomer, as it is only possible to correct the error by reading the creator's mind. Error *recovery* is perhaps a better word. At any rate, repairing the error may allow the parser to continue finding errors. It may also cause it to find spurious, nonexistent errors.

Consulting one or more of the references in the selected reading or the documentation for whatever tool you are using or devising a method of your own, add syntactic error handling to your generated parser. Run your error-handling parser on:

(a) ```
begun
    a := b3 ;
    xyz := a + b + c
                - p / q ;
    a = xyz * (p + q);
    p := a - xyz - p ;
end.
```

(b) ```
begin
    if i > j then ;
    i := i + j ;
    elsif i < j then ;
    i := 1 ;
    end of ;
    end ;
```

(c) ```
begin
    while (i < j) and (j < k loop
    k := k + 1 ;
    while (i = j) loop ;
    i := i + 2 ;
    end loop ;
end ;
```

(d) The empty program

(e) A program of your choice

## Part IV

## Abstract Syntax Trees

This assignment can be done following the material in Chapter 6. Students report times of 15–20 hours for this assignment.

Define a set of abstract syntax tree nodes for the language which your compiler currently implements. Add attributes and semantic functions to perform this translation:

```
        plus
       ╱    ╲
  opnd1    opnd2
```

is an AST node for $a + b$ where a is opnd1 and b is opnd2. In parenthesized form, this could be written:

```
(plus ("a" "b"))  or  (+ ("a" "b"))
```

Two of the productions that relate to such a node are:

```
...
Relation            →  SimpleExpression
SimpleExpression    →  Term₁ {AddingOperator Term₂}
...
```
```

(The dots represent the productions which come before and after these two.)
    If we create a data structure:

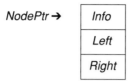

then we can add attributes such as the following:

```
. . .
Relation          →  SimpleExpression
                     Relation.NodePtr = SimpleExpression.NodePtr
SimpleExpression  →  Term₁ {AddingOperator Term₂}
                     SimpleExpression.NodePtr := {GetNode}
                     SimpleExpression.Info := "+"
                     SimpleExpression.Left := Term₁.NodePtr
                     SimpleExpression..Right := Term₂.NodePtr
```

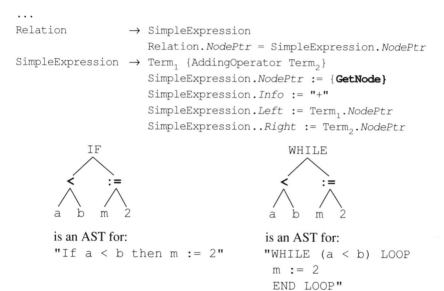

is an AST for:
"If a < b then m := 2"

is an AST for:
"WHILE (a < b) LOOP
   m := 2
 END LOOP"

In parenthesized form these might be written:

```
(IF  ("<"  ("a"  "b")  ":="  ("m"  "2")))  and
(WHILE  ("<"  ("a"  "b")  ":="  (":="  ("m"  "2")))
```

Attributes and semantic functions may be added analogously to those of the "+" node
above. Indenting will make the AST easier to read.

    Design attributes and semantic functions which will translate your programs to
abstract syntax trees. Add semantic actions to whatever tool you are using to translate input programs to AST's. Most tools do not allow the attribute grammar syntax,
so the semantic functions should be implemented in the way which your tool expects.
Print them out in parenthesized form.

    If your tool allows attribute grammar descriptions, then you may be able to trans-
late your attribute grammar directly. Run your program with all the preceding programs. (You need no longer print out tokens and parse information.)

Part V

Symbol Tables

Students report times **in excess** of 25 hours for this assignment.

1. Add a symbol table to your program. Define its structure and a compiler switch to allow the printing of the symbol table after compilation.

2. Enhance your program to scan and parse programs described by the grammar of the previous assignment with the addition of declarations and array features as described by the following BNF.

3. Write your routines which access the symbol table as *abstract functions* and *procedures*, that is, the calling procedures, e.g.,

```
enter(SymbolTable,Name)
```

needn't know what the symbol table looks like.

4. Print by name in alphabetical order.

5. Your symbol table should contain attributes for class, line numbers, and scoping (the enhancement assignment adds procedures and functions). The following shows a program excerpt and the corresponding symbol table entries.

Input Program

```
. . .
List : Array [1..100] of integer ;
a : Integer;
. . .
BEGIN
. . . .
END
```

Symbol Table

Name	Class	Scope	Definition Line No.	Reference Line Nos.	Other
...					
a	Integer	0	#		
...					
List	Array of Integer	0	#	#, #, #	One Dimensional
...					

NEW BNF (Merge with old BNF)

Program	→	DeclarativePart
		begin
		SequenceOfStatements
		end;
DeclarativePart	→	{BasicDeclarativeItem}
BasicDeclarativeItem	→	BasicDeclaration

```
BasicDeclaration            →  ObjectDeclaration
ObjectDeclaration           →  IdentifierList : SubtypeIndication;
SubtypeIndication           →  TypeDefinition | TypeMark
TypeDefinition              →  ArrayTypeDefinition
ArrayTypeDefinition         →  ConstrainedArrayDefinition
ConstrainedArrayDefinition  →  array [ConstrainedIndexList] of
                                  ElementType
ConstrainedIndexList        →  DiscreteRange {, DiscreteRange}
DiscreteRange               →  Range
Range                       →  SimpleExpression .. SimpleExpression
ElementType                 →  TypeMark
TypeMark                    →  integer | boolean
IdentifierList              →  Identifier {, Identifier}
name                        →  SimpleName | SimpleName {NameSuffix}
NameSuffix                  →  (Expression {, Expression})
```

Part VI

(Optional) Enhancement

Add functions and procedures to your program. The following syntax describes function and procedure declarations and calls. It should be merged with the previous BNF's. *Compilation* becomes the new start symbol of the grammar.

```
Compilation               →  {CompilationUnit}
CompilationUnit           →  SubprogramBody
ActualParameter           →  Expression | Name
ActualParameterPart       →  (ParameterAssociation {, ParameterAsso-
                                ciation})
FormalPart                →  (ParameterSpecification {; Parameter-
                                Specification})
FunctionCall              →  Name [ActualParameterPart]
Mode                      →  in | inout | out
ParameterAssociation      →  ActualParameter
ParameterSpecification    →  IdentifierList : Mode TypeMark
Primary                   →  FunctionCall
ProcedureCallStatement    →  Name [ActualParameterPart] ;
ReturnStatement           →  return Expression ;
SimpleStatement           →  ProcedureCallStatement
SubprogramBody            →  SubprogramSpecification is [Declara-
                                tivePart]
                             begin
                                SequenceOfStatements
                             end ;
SubprogramSpecification   →  procedure Identifier [FormalPart]
                             function Identifier [FormalPart] return
                                                                TypeMark
```

Part VII

Code Generation

Although the amount of time will vary according to how much the student implements, typical times reported are around 20 hours.

1. Write a simple code generator for the Ada subset you have implemented.
   (a) You should also do some *simple* register allocation. Be sure to describe your method clearly.
   (b) You MUST translate from the intermediate representation (the AST and the symbol table). Do not add actions to your grammar to produce code.
   (c) You may translate it into any assembly language, but if you know the assembly language for the machine you are using, that is preferable.

   Hints: (1) Start by generating code for assignment statements, adding other constructs one at a time. (2) A simple *working* code generator is better that an elaborate *non-working* one!!! You may never get embedded procedures or even WHILE's and IF's working.

2. Run your compiler on various programs. Output should be the assembly language code. If you are on the machine that uses your assembly language, assemble and run (perhaps using the debugger) and hand in something that shows your code executing correctly. This is the final assignment. Package and document it well!

3. Assemble and run your code. Convince yourself (and your instructor) that it works.

4. Include documentation describing your language. Be sure to include the BNF for the subset of Ada which your program compiles.

Index

Abstract syntax tree, 230
Action, 25–26
    of parser driver for LR-family, 75–76
Action symbol, 100
Activation records
    and block structure, 255–257
    and concurrent units, 259
    and recursion, 254–255
    and storage management, 252, 258–259
    and unit activation, 255–257
Ada, 17, 21, 33, 250, 265–266
Addressing mode, 239
Algebraic identities, 193–194
Algorithms, and optimization, 143–144
Array, 84, 204, 231–232, 261–263
Array processors, 275–276
Attribute, 11, 95
    inherited, 96, 101, 107
    intrinsic, 97
    synthesized, 96, 101, 107
Attribute evaluation, 106–117, 264
    and complexity, 106–117
    and dependency graphs, 106–117
    and dynamic sequence evaluator, 108–112
    and method of Katayama, 106–117
    and method of Ramanathan and Kennedy, 106–117
    of PSOOL, 122–124
    symbol tables, 117–119
Attribute grammar, 3, 25, 32, 95, 96, 104, 120, 262–263, 264
    absolutely noncircular, 104–105, 106
    definition of, 11
    and implementing the semantics of PSOOL, 119–124
    noncircular, 102
Attributes of PSOOL, 120–121
Automata, 42–47
Available expressions, 165, 169–173
    computing, 169–172
    use of, 173
Axiomatic semantics, 24

Back edge, 158
Backpatching, 150
Backus-Naur form, 3, 56, 248
    for PSOOL, 21–24
Backwards edge, and natural loops, 160
Backwards flow, and data flow analysis, 165
Basic blocks, 147–148, 150, 192
Benchmark, 250
Binding, 20, 252
Block, and symbol tables, 117
Block structured language, 118, 255–257
BNF, see Backus-Naur form
Bottom-up parser generator, 73–93
    error handling in LR-family parsing, 83–84
    LR-family parsing, 75–83
    metalanguage, 74–75
    table representation and compaction, 84
    YACC, 84–87
Branches, 240

C, 17, 21, 274
Cactus stack, 259
Case, 63
Cattell, method of, for table-driven code generation, 236–237
Circularity, 102
CISC, 271
    and debugging optimized code, 274
Class, 20, 21, 27–29
    and object-oriented languages, 19
    and symbol tables, 117–118
Class descriptions, 27–32
ClassName, as attribute in PSOOL compiler, 120
Code generation, 14, 95, 223–246
    from DAGs, 234–235
    as feature of production-quality compilers, 249
    instruction selection from IRs, 229–233
    phase, 223
    phases of
        code selection, 223
        peephole optimization, 223, 239–242
        preparation for, 223

305